D0009298

O A E L

OXFORD AMERICAN ENDOCRINOLOGY LIBRARY

Diabetes: Improving Patient Care

DATE DUE

This material is not intended to be, and should not be considered, a substitut for medical or other professional advice. Treatment for the conditions describe in this material is highly dependent on the individual circumstances. While thi material is designed to offer accurate information with respect to the subjec matter covered and to be current as of the time it was written, research an knowledge about medical and health issues are constantly evolving, and dos schedules for medications are being revised continually, with new side effects rec ognized and accounted for regularly. Readers must therefore always check th product information and clinical procedures with the most up-to-date publishe product information and data sheets provided by the manufacturers and the mos recent codes of conduct and safety regulation. Oxford University Press and th authors make no representations or warranties to readers, express or implied, a to the accuracy or completeness of this material, including without limitation tha they make no representations or warranties as to the accuracy or efficacy of th drug dosages mentioned in the material. The authors and the publishers do nc accept, and expressly disclaim, any responsibility for any liability, loss, or risk tha may be claimed or incurred as a consequence of the use and/or application of an of the contents of this material.

O A E L
OXFORD AMERICAN ENDOCRINOLOGY LIBRARY

Diabetes: Improving Patient Care

Vivian Fonseca, MD

Professor of Medicine and Pharmacology
Tullis–Tulane Alumni Chair in Diabetes
Chief, Section of Endocrinology
Tulane University Health Sciences Center
New Orleans, LA

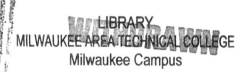

OXFORD
UNIVERSITY PRESS
2010

OXFORD
UNIVERSITY PRESS

Oxford University Press, Inc., publishes works that further
Oxford University's objective of excellence
in research, scholarship, and education.

Oxford New York
Auckland Cape Town Dar es Salaam Hong Kong Karachi
Kuala Lumpur Madrid Melbourne Mexico City Nairobi
New Delhi Shanghai Taipei Toronto

With offices in
Argentina Austria Brazil Chile Czech Republic France Greece
Guatemala Hungary Italy Japan Poland Portugal Singapore
South Korea Switzerland Thailand Turkey Ukraine Vietnam

Copyright © 2010 by Oxford University Press, Inc.

Published by Oxford University Press, Inc.
198 Madison Avenue, New York, New York 10016
www.oup.com

Oxford is a registered trademark of Oxford University Press

Library of Congress Cataloging-in-Publication Data

Diabetes: improving patient care/[edited by] Vivian Fonseca.
p. ; cm.—(Oxford American psychiatry library)
Includes bibliographical references.
ISBN 978-0-19-538211-2
1. Diabetes—Treatment. I. Fonseca, Vivian A. II. Series.
[DNLM: 1. Diabetes Mellitus—therapy. 2. Diabetes Mellitus—diagnosis.
3. Diabetes Mellitus—prevention & control. 4. Insulin—therapeutic use.
5. Life Style. 6. Self Care. WK 815 D53554 2008]
RC660.D447 2008
616.4'62—dc22   2008034981

Printed in the United States of America
on acid-free paper

Preface

We face an unprecedented epidemic of diabetes and obesity that threatens to afflict a large segment of the population and decrease life expectancy as well as quality of life. Furthermore, although we have made tremendous advances in treatment, it appears that we cannot achieve normal blood sugars safely in high-risk patients.

Clinicians face many challenges in dealing with the epidemic. Efficient strategies must be developed to evaluate and treat large numbers of patients and to motivate patients to understand the underlying problems, to change their lifestyle, and to comply with complex treatment regimens.

In this book, we have attempted to offer practical advice on how to evaluate patients and treat them effectively, from the first visit to the late-stage patient with complications.

I am delighted to have eminent colleagues join me in this endeavor. Guillermo Umpierrez has particular expertise in patient evaluation and in effective strategies for insulin use. Richard Rubin and Mark Peyrot have pioneered studies to improve patients' motivation and hence compliance with treatment and lifestyle change. Finally, Susie Villalobos offers practical advice on diabetes education and diet, which can be accomplished in any clinical setting.

I hope that you will find this book useful and that it will stimulate you to improve the care of your patients with diabetes. I would like to dedicate the book to those with diabetes who were impacted by Hurricane Katrina and who are still struggling to adjust, in its aftermath, to the complexities of this disease.

Vivian Fonseca

Contributors

Guillermo E. Umpierrez, MD

Professor of Medicine
Emory University School
    of Medicine
Atlanta, GA

Susie Wiegert Villalobos, MPH, LDN, RD

Program Coordinator/Dietitian
    Tulane Center for Diabetes/
    Endocrine Weight Management
    Program
Tulane Medical Center—Lakeside
    Campus
New Orleans, LA

Richard R. Rubin, PhD

Professor, Medicine
    and Pediatrics
The Johns Hopkins
    University School of
    Medicine
Baltimore, MD

Mark Peyrot, PhD

Department of Sociology
Loyola College
Department of Medicine
The Johns Hopkins University
    School of Medicine
Baltimore, MD

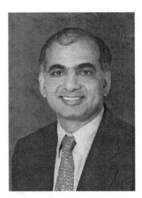

Vivian Fonseca
Tulane University Medical Center
New Orleans, Louisiana, USA

Vivian Fonseca, MD, MRCP, is Professor of Medicine, the Tullis–Tulane Alumni Chair in Diabetes, and chief of the Section of Endocrinology at Tulane University Medical Center in New Orleans, Louisiana. He is a fellow of the American Association of Clinical Endocrinologists, the Royal College of Physicians, London, UK, and the American College of Physicians. Dr. Fonseca has previously been editor-in-chief of the *Journal of the Metabolic Syndrome and Related Disorders* and served on the editorial board of the *Journal of Clinical Endocrinology and Metabolism* (2003–2006). He has been editor-in-chief of *Diabetes Care* since 2007, having formerly been associate editor, and is an ad hoc reviewer for several other journals, including *New England Journal of Medicine, Journal of the American Medical Association, Diabetes, Diabetic Medicine, Kidney International, The American Journal of Clinical Nutrition, British Medical Journal,* and *Metabolism.*

Dr. Fonseca's current research interests include the prevention and treatment of diabetic complications and risk factor reduction in cardiovascular disease. He has a research program evaluating homocysteine and inflammation as risk factors for heart disease in diabetes and is also an investigator in the NIH-funded Action to Control Cardiovascular Risk in Diabetes (ACCORD) study. He is co-investigator on the NIH TINSAL-2D study and serves on the Steering and Ancillary Studies Committees and Glycemia Control Committee. Dr. Fonseca is also an investigator on "The Impact of Hurricane Katrina on Diabetes and Co-morbidities." He is a member of the Board of Directors of the American Diabetes Association (ADA) and the national Leadership Council and is president of the Louisiana Leadership Council of the ADA. Dr. Fonseca has served on various ADA committees such as the Professional Practice and Research Policy Committees, as well as the joint ADA/ACC "Make the Link" Program. He is also a member of the Endocrine Society and the International Diabetes Federation. Dr. Fonseca has published over 200 papers, review articles, monographs, and book chapters and is editor of the textbook *Clinical Diabetes: Translating Research into Practice.*

Contents

Chapter 1

Meeting goals in diabetes—why and how

Vivian Fonseca

Diabetes mellitus (DM) has emerged as one of the most serious global health care problems. The estimated number of people with DM worldwide in 2000 was 171 million and is expected to increase to 366 million by 2030. In addition, approximately 197 million people worldwide have impaired glucose tolerance (IGT), a prediabetic state; this number is expected to increase to 420 million by 2025. Of great concern is the fact that the highest increase in the number of diabetics is projected to occur in developing countries, where the number of people with DM is expected to increase by three-fold. In the United States, more than 20 million individuals (over 7% of the population) have DM, and in addition more than 40 million have IGT or prediabetes. The incidences of both type 1 and type 2 DM (T1DM and T2DM, respectively) are increasing, and they often occur in the setting of obesity, making treatment challenging. Many abnormalities associated with obesity tend to cluster in patients with T2DM, resulting in an increased risk of not only the microvascular complications of DM but also excess cardiovascular disease.

DM is a highly prevalent public health problem, having reached epidemic status worldwide. It contributes greatly to morbidity and mortality in a large segment of the population, and, due to its expensive complications, it is a great burden on health care systems. The prevalence of DM varies considerably and is closely linked to obesity, but in some populations a strong genetic predisposition leads to high prevalence rates. Examples of the latter include American Indians, African Americans, and Latinos, particularly those living in the United States, and Asian Indians, with a considerable increase in the prevalence of the condition in countries such as India over the past decade.

The main purpose of this book is to identify practical strategies to get people to reach and maintain their therapeutic goals in order to prevent complications. It is therefore appropriate that we should first consider the goals for DM management outlined in Figure 1.1.

The primary goal of treating glycemia is to reduce the Hb_{A1c} to a level where the risk of complications is significantly reduced without a risk of serious side effects. Data suggest that this is accomplished for microvascular complications of DM (see Chapter 5) at an Hb_{A1c} of <7%. However, for cardiovascular events, such as myocardial infarction, the relationship

- Glycemia—goal A1C <7% (as close to normal [<6%] as possible in individual patients)
- Hypertension—goal <130/80 mm Hg
- Dyslipidemia
  - —goal LDL-C <100 mg/dL* (<70 mg/dL an option in high cardiovascular [CV] risk patients)
  - —goal HDL-C—men >40 mg/dL; women >50 mg/dL
  - —goal TGs <150 mg/dL
- Prothrombotic state—aspirin Rx (75 to 162 mg/day) in adult patients with diabetes and CVD or for primary prevention in patients >40 years with diabetes and >1 other CV risk factor(s)
- Cigarette smoking goal—cessation

Figure 1.1 ADA Goals for Diabetes Management—2008. *Source:* American Diabetes Association. Standards of Medical Care in Diabetes—2008. *Diabetes Care.* 31: S12–54S. Reprinted with permission of the American Diabetes Association.
*If drug-treated patients do not reach target on maximal tolerated statin therapy, consider an LDL-C reduction of ~40% from baseline as an alternative therapeutic goal.

with Hb_{A1c} is not linear and other factors such as lipids and blood pressure (BP) are important. The relationship between Hb_{A1c} and microvascular/macrovascular complications in the UK Prospective Diabetes Study trial[1] is illustrated in Figure 5.1 (see Chapter 5).

The goals and strategies for managing T1DM evolved from the Diabetes Control and Complications Trial (DCCT),[2] which clearly demonstrated both the value and risks associated with good glycemic control. Our approach to the treatment of T2DM has gradually evolved over the past few years to include a "holistic" approach that addresses lifestyle change and treatment of multiple risk factors and also addresses many treatment targets that involve the pathophysiology of the condition, as well as attempts to halt or slow the progression of the disease. Table 1.1 summarizes some of the newer concepts in treating T2DM.

Pathophysiology

The pathophysiology of DM is complex and is dependent on the type of DM, as described later. The differences between the types of DM are highlighted in Table 1.2.

Type 1 diabetes

T1DM is characterized by an absolute deficiency of insulin. Because insulin has a major action on adipose tissue formation and breakdown, deficiency of insulin leads to increased ketone body production and ketoacidosis. A history of ketoacidosis is used as the important defining feature of T1DM.[3] It is generally thought that T1DM is an autoimmune disorder with antibodies that destroy pancreatic β cells and that it is frequently associated with other antibodies and other autoimmune processes in the body (thyroid autoimmunity, etc.). However, in a few patients, ketoacidosis may

Table 1.1 Newer and evolving concepts in treating diabetes

- Lifestyle change for prevention (as well as treatment)
- Pharmacological therapy (metformin) at diagnosis and possibly prevention
- Early combination therapy
- Overcome barriers to earlier insulin use
- Aggressive multiple risk factor reduction
- Preferentially targeting postprandial glucose at lower Hb_{A1c} levels
- Halting disease progression

Table 1.2 Differentiating type 1 and type 2 diabetes

Classic features of type 1 diabetes
- History of ketoacidosis/ketonuria
- Weight loss at diagnosis
- Often severe symptoms
- Dependency on insulin—ketosis if insulin is missed
- Islet cell antibodies early, GAD antibodies persist
- Late-onset type 1 has slower onset—associated with GAD antibody
- Low or undetectable C-peptide
- Other autoimmune disorders (eg. hypothyroidism)

Classic features suggesting type 2 diabetes
- Positive family history
- Ethnic origin—African American, Latino, American Indian
- History of gestational diabetes, polycystic ovary syndrome
- Obesity
- Acanthosis nigricans

not be associated with classic T1DM and may represent a transient absolute deficiency of β-cell function in patients who otherwise have classic T2DM. In addition, some patients with typical T1DM have neither identifiable autoimmune disease nor detectable antibodies. Nevertheless, such patients are classified as having T1DM and are treated as such with insulin therapy.

T1DM was classically described as having an onset in childhood and is associated with a lean body habitus. However, it has been recently recognized that many children with DM indeed have T2DM due to obesity in childhood and, conversely, some patients with the onset of DM later in life actually have T1DM.

There has been a gradual increase in the incidence of T1DM, and hypotheses to explain this increase include an increase in viral illness precipitating autoimmunity and obesity accelerating inflammation and autoimmune phenomena, among others.

Can we predict T1DM and detect it early? Several T1DM prevention studies have helped identify people at risk, usually by testing siblings of patients. Predictors include certain HLA types (DR3 and DR4), the presence of islet cell antibodies and other antibodies, etc. However, the value of predicting T1DM is small because currently no preventive strategy has proved to be effective. However, in selected cases, it may help identify patients with surveillance, so that treatment can be started early before the patient develops the crisis state of ketoacidosis.

Type 2 diabetes

T2DM is a very common disorder, with over 7% of the general population having the condition, and almost half of them are unaware of the diagnosis due to its slow onset. It is frequently associated with obesity and aging but, in recent years, has been frequently seen in children and adolescents who are obese.

T2DM is characterized by multiple pathophysiological abnormalities, including an underlying insulin resistance, which may be present for many years before the onset of DM. DM in such individuals is prevented by an increase in pancreatic insulin production, and it is only when the pancreas fails to produce enough insulin and there is a relative insulin deficiency that DM becomes clinically manifest by its current definition. Thus, there are at least two abnormalities characteristic of classic DM—insulin resistance and pancreatic β-cell dysfunction leading to relative insulin deficiency. The insulin deficiency is further characterized as lacking rapid response of the β cell to a rise in glucose—called first-phase insulin secretion. This abnormality occurs very early in the natural history of DM and contributes to IGT and postprandial hyperglycemia.

In addition, other abnormalities have been identified, such as an excess of glucagon secretion, particularly lack of suppression of glucagon after a meal, which leads to increased production of glucose in the liver and postprandial hyperglycemia. In addition, there appear to be deficiencies of some gastrointestinal hormones, called incretins, which may contribute to lack of suppression of glucagon.[4] Finally, amylin, a pancreatic hormone that is normally co-secreted with insulin, may contribute to glucose homeostasis, particularly in advanced T2DM. Its secretion appears to be diminished in advanced T2DM, but its action is preserved. Amylin has been found to slow gastric emptying, suppress postprandial glucagon secretion, and increase satiety.

The pathophysiology of hyperglycemia is thus very complex, with more than one abnormality being present in most patients. In the natural history of the disease, insulin resistance usually appears very early and is commonly associated with obesity. This can be compensated for by increased pancreatic insulin secretion, which may persist for many years before pancreatic failure sets in. At that stage, overt clinical DM becomes manifest. Pancreatic endocrine function then continues to decline despite therapy, necessitating additional steps to therapy. Recent data suggest that the rate of failure may vary with different types of treatment,[5] creating an opportunity to select therapies more likely to succeed in the long term.

There are multiple facets to the above-mentioned abnormalities. For example, insulin resistance may occur in the liver as well as in muscle and adipose tissue, necessitating the use of different drugs that target insulin sensitivity in these various tissues and can be used in combination (metformin and thiazolidinediones, respectively). Similarly, multiple defects have been described in the pancreatic islet in response to meal challenges and carbohydrate load (e.g., decreased insulin and amylin and increased glucagon), resulting in new targets for treatment. Not only is insulin secretion reduced, particularly in relation to meals, but also increased gluconeogenesis and excess hepatic glucose production have been identified as important pathophysiological abnormalities that can now be corrected.

There is increasing evidence that the incretin system also may play a role in glucose homeostasis.[4] The incretin hormone most strongly implicated is glucagon-like peptide 1 (GLP-1). GLP-1 is a naturally occurring peptide produced by the L cells of the small intestine. Although GLP-1 secretion is reduced in patients with T2DM, its action is preserved. GLP-1 enhances glucose-dependent insulin secretion, suppresses hepatic glucagon secretion, slows gastric emptying, and increases satiety. In normal conditions, GLP-1 is very rapidly cleaved and inactivated by the enzyme dipeptidyl peptidase IV (DPP-IV), which makes native GLP-1 impractical for use as a DM treatment. However, other strategies to prolong GLP-1 action, including GLP-1 analogues resistant to DPP-IV inactivation and inhibitors of DPP-IV (see later section), have been developed as antihyperglycemic agents.

Because β-cell failure is progressive in T2DM, treatment interventions must be continuously monitored and advanced, with stepwise addition of noninsulin agents and/or insulin over time. An agent that could halt the decline in β-cell function, therefore, would be of tremendous benefit. An approach to address these underlying problems would therefore include the use of medications to reduce insulin resistance and improve pancreatic function. Therapy directed at both these abnormalities is frequently used in combination.

Gestational diabetes

Gestational diabetes mellitus (GDM) is defined as any degree of glucose intolerance with onset or first recognition during pregnancy. GDM is a major health problem in the United States. It affects 5% to 7% of all pregnancies and is associated with increased maternal and perinatal morbidity. Approximately 7% of all pregnancies (ranging from 1% to 14% depending on the population studied and the diagnostic tests used) are complicated by GDM, amounting to more than 200,000 cases annually. Women with GDM are also at increased risk of subsequently developing overt DM. Several potentially reversible risk factors for GDM have been identified, including obesity, elevated plasma glucose in the fasting state, and sedentary lifestyle.

GDM occurs as a result of a combination of insulin resistance and diminished insulin secretion. Human studies have estimated a reduction in insulin sensitivity of 50% to 60% during pregnancy.[6]

Fasting plasma insulin increases gradually during a normal pregnancy to reach levels that are approximately twice as high in the third trimester as the levels outside pregnancy. In the face of exaggerated insulin resistance, women with GDM have reduced pancreatic β-cell function during late pregnancy compared with normal pregnant women. This reduction has been estimated to be in the range of 34% to 41% based on simple comparisons of first-phase insulin responses to intravenous glucose and early insulin responses to oral glucose between normal pregnant and GDM groups.

Because of the risks of GDM to the mother and neonate, screening and diagnosis are warranted. The screening and diagnostic strategies are based on the American Diabetes Association position statement on GDM. Because women with a history of GDM have a greatly increased subsequent risk for DM, they should be screened for DM 6 to 12 weeks postpartum, using standard criteria, and should be followed up with subsequent screening for the development of DM or prediabetes.

Prediabetes

Table 1.3 outlines the diagnostic criteria for DM. The term "prediabetes" has come back into recognition in the past few years due to development of strategies to prevent DM. It encompasses both IGT (glucose 140 to 199 mg/dL at 2 hours during a 75 g oral glucose tolerance test) and impaired fasting glucose (fasting blood glucose 100 to 125 mg/dL). The importance of recognizing prediabetes is that a large number of patients will progress over time to DM unless intervention strategies are implemented. In addition, prediabetes clusters with a number of other cardiovascular risk factors, such as high blood pressure, elevated triglycerides and low HDL cholesterol, and central obesity. The term "metabolic syndrome" is sometimes used in the diagnosis and characterization of such patients who are clearly at increased risk of future cardiovascular disease. Intervention strategies in such patients should therefore include not only prevention of DM but also prevention of cardiovascular disease.

Screening for diabetes—who should be screened for diabetes and prediabetes?

Table 1.4 outlines patient groups at high risk for future development of DM and who may be appropriate targets for screening below the age of 45. Above the age of 45, all persons should have a fasting blood test, repeated every 3 years as long as it is normal.

Table 1.3 Criteria for the diagnosis of diabetes

Any one of the following:

1. Symptoms of diabetes (polyuria, polydipsia, unexplained weight loss) plus random plasma glucose concentration 200 mg/dL (11.1 mmol/L).

2. FPG >126 mg/dL (7.0 mmol/L) (fasting = no caloric intake for at least 8 hours)

3. 2-hour plasma glucose 200 mg/dL during an oral glucose tolerance test (OGTT) (75 g)

In the absence of unequivocal hyperglycemia with acute metabolic decompensation, these criteria should be confirmed by repeat testing on a different day.

Table 1.4 Who should be screened for diabetes

Consider testing for all individuals >45 years; if normal, repeat every 3 years.

Consider testing at a younger age or more frequently for high-risk individuals:

- Obese (>120% desirable body weight or a BMI >27 kg/m^2)
- Having a first-degree relative with diabetes
- Member of a high-risk ethnic population (e.g., African American, Hispanic, Native American)
- Delivered a baby weighing >9 lb or has been diagnosed with gestational diabetes mellitus
- Hypertensive (>140/90 mm Hg)
- Having an HDL-C level >35 mg/dL and/or a triglyceride level >250 mg/dL
- History of polycystic ovary syndrome or fatty liver
- Impaired glucose tolerance or impaired fasting glycemia on previous testing

Table 1.5 Strategies for the prevention of diabetes

- Patients with impaired glucose tolerance or impaired fasting glycemia should be given counseling on weight loss of 5% to 10% of body weight, as well as on increasing physical activity to at least 150 min/week of moderate activity such as walking.
- Follow-up counseling appears to be important for success.
- In addition to lifestyle counseling, metformin may be considered in those who are at very high risk (impaired glucose tolerance or impaired fasting glycemia plus other risk factors) and who are obese and <60 years of age.
- Monitoring for the development of diabetes in those with prediabetes should be performed every year.

Noninvasive screening tools have recently been developed to identify people at risk for undiagnosed DM and prediabetes.[7] Such patients should also undergo frequent screening.

Strategies in prevention of DM in patients with prediabetes (Table 1.5) should follow the model of DM prevention program with encouragement of weight loss of about 5% for calorie restriction and increasing physical activity to at least brisk walking for 30 minutes every day. In addition, in selected patients it may be appropriate to consider the use of metformin, particularly for patients who continue to progress despite lifestyle change. However, this use of metformin is not approved by the U.S. Food and Drug Administration.

Overcoming the problem

Several studies have given us tools to help alleviate the burden of DM by preventing both the onset of the disease and its complications. These include landmark studies like the DCCT, UKPDS, and STENO-2.[8,9] On the other hand, some caution is needed in attempting normoglycemia, as this may increase risk for patients, as seen in the ACCORD study.[10] Nevertheless, the ADVANCE study showed that reducing Hb$_{A1c}$ to <6.5% led to a decrease in the composite of microvascular and macrovascular

Table 1.6 Lessons from clinical trials

Lessons from clinical trials in type 1 diabetes

- Multiple daily injections or pump therapy is needed to get most patients to goal.
- Frequent monitoring or continuous glucose monitoring system is needed.
- Hypoglycemia is a major barrier to achieving goals.
- Complications may transiently worsen before patients improve.
- Intensive treatment is associated with improved quality of life despite increased injections/monitoring and hypoglycemia.

Lessons from clinical trials in type 2 diabetes

- It is difficult to achieve normoglycemia.
- Attempting normoglycemia may be associated with increased risk of hypoglycemia and all cause mortality in some patients.
- Lifestyle change is important but is not sufficient to control blood glucose once diabetes is diagnosed.
- Monotherapy usually fails over time.
- The rate failure of drug therapy varies across different medications.
- Cardiovascular disease in diabetes remains a major clinical challenge.
- Sulfonylureas have a high failure rate over 4 to 5 years—there is less failure with metformin and thiazolidinediones.
- Insulin therapy is usually required in long-term diabetes mellitus.

Table 1.7 Summary of strategies to achieve goals

1. Early diagnosis and treatment
2. Diabetes education—must be frequently reinforced
3. Early combination treatment—lower doses in combination may minimize side effects
4. Do not delay insulin use
5. Institute multiple risk factor reduction—A1c, BP, Lipids, aspirin
6. Frequent clinic visits
7. Address nonadherence to therapy (motivation, depression, etc.)

events, without increasing mortality—perhaps because a less aggressive treatment approach was used.[11] Thus, reducing Hb_{A1c} to <7% will clearly reduce the risk of microvascular events and have some, albeit small, impact on cardiovascular disease events. To reduce the latter, we should clearly focus on optimal control of blood pressure and lipids, while keeping the blood glucose at a level that does not increase risk. These strategies are outlined in Tables 1.6 through 1.7 and discussed further in Chapter 5.[7] The details of the individual strategies using lifestyle change and medication are discussed in subsequent chapters.

References

1. Stratton IM, Adler AI, Neil HA, et al. Association of glycaemia with macrovascular and microvascular complications of type 2 diabetes (UKPDS 35): prospective observational study. *BMJ.* 2000;321:405–412.

2. Effect of intensive therapy on the microvascular complications of type 1 diabetes mellitus. *JAMA*. 2002;287:2563–2569.

3. American Diabetes Association. Standards of medical care in diabetes—2008. *Diabetes Care*. 2008;31 Suppl 1:S12–S54.

4. Drucker DJ. The role of gut hormones in glucose homeostasis. *J Clin Invest*. 2007;117:24–32.

5. Kahn SE, Haffner SM, Heise MA, et al. Glycemic durability of rosiglitazone, metformin, or glyburide monotherapy. *N Engl J Med*. 2006;355:2427–2443.

6. Lain KY, Catalano PM. Metabolic changes in pregnancy. *Clin Obstet Gynecol*. 2007;50:938–948.

7. Heikes KE, Eddy DM, Arondekar B, Schlessinger L. Diabetes risk calculator: a simple tool for detecting undiagnosed diabetes and prediabetes. *Diabetes Care*. 2008;31:1040–1045.

8. Gaede P, Lund-Andersen H, Parving HH, Pedersen O. Effect of a multifactorial intervention on mortality in type 2 diabetes. *N Engl J Med*. 2008;358:580–591.

9. UK Prospective Diabetes Study (UKPDS) Group. Intensive blood-glucose control with sulphonylureas or insulin compared with conventional treatment and risk of complications in patients with type 2 diabetes (UKPDS 33). *Lancet*. 1998;352:837–853.

10. Action to Control Cardiovascular Risk in Diabetes Study Group, Gerstein HC, Miller ME, et al. Effects of intensive glucose lowering in type 2 diabetes. *N Engl J Med*. 2008;358:2545–2559.

11. The ADVANCE Collaborative Group. Intensive blood glucose control and vascular outcomes in patients with type 2 diabetes. *N Engl J Med*. 2008;358:2560–2572.

Chapter 2

The office visit: Setting the goals

Guillermo E. Umpierrez

The proper care of a patient with diabetes requires a team approach led by a physician and including diabetes educators, nurses, physician assistants, dietitians, pharmacists, and mental health professionals. The diabetes team should provide specific nutrition, exercise, and pharmacological recommendations as well as diabetes self-management education (DSME). This chapter aims to review standards of care and practice guidelines that apply to adult patients.

A comprehensive clinical valuation should be performed during the initial visit. It is important to determine the type and duration of diabetes and to review previous treatment and level of glycemic control in order to formulate the management plan.[1] Medical evaluation should be performed to detect the presence of hypertension, cardiovascular disease (CVD), and microvascular complications. Recommended clinical and diagnostic tests for the evaluation of a patient with diabetes are included in Table 2.1.

Diabetes self-management education

The aims of DSME are to provide patients with the knowledge and skills necessary to achieve optimal control of their diabetes and to assist them in becoming effective, self-directed decision makers for their own diabetes care.[2] Patient education should be provided at every opportunity of encounter with the patient and his or her family, and either the education should be conducted in the physician's office or the patient should be referred to a facility or organization certified by the American Diabetes Association (ADA) or American Association of Diabetes Educators (AADE). It cannot be overstated that a well-informed patient (regardless of the level of education) is essential for good diabetes care. To be successful, the diabetes education program should be easy to understand, at a low-literacy level. A good-quality DSME program shall offer a diabetes overview; nutrition, exercise, and activity recommendations; indications and use of glucose-monitoring devices; prevention, detection, and treatment of acute and chronic diabetic complications; foot, skin, and dental care; benefits, risks, and management options for improving diabetes control; and, if indicated,

Table 2.1 Recommended periodic medical assessment, laboratory tests, counseling, and education in patients with diabetes

History and physical examination	Recommended frequency
Blood pressure	Every 3 to 6 months
Height and weight, BMI	Every 3 to 6 months
Dilated eye examination	T1DM: after 3 to 5 years of diagnosis, then annually
	T2DM: shortly after diagnosis, then annually
Foot examination	Every 3 to 6 months
Lower extremity sensory examination	Initial/annual
Dental examination	Every 6 months
Laboratory tests	
Hb_{A1c}	Every 3 to 6 months
Urine microalbumin	Initial/annual
Serum creatinine/calculated GFR	Initial/annual
Fasting lipid profile	Initial/annual
Thyroid-stimulating hormone	Initial/as indicated
Counseling/education	
Review self-management skills	Initial/ongoing
Screen for depression	Initial/annual
Smoking status	Initial/ongoing

a smoking cessation program and review of preconception care, pregnancy, and gestational diabetes (Table 2.2).

Assessment of glycemic control

Specific goals for glycemic control are the same for adult subjects with type 1 diabetes mellitus (T1DM) and those with type 2 diabetes mellitus (T2DM). Two tests are recommended in assessing glycemic control: patient self-monitoring of blood glucose (SMBG) and Hb_{A1c} measurement. SMBG is especially important for patients treated with insulin or sulfonylureas to monitor for and prevent asymptomatic hypoglycemia and extreme hyperglycemia.[1] Patients with T1DM and those with T2DM receiving insulin therapy should monitor their blood glucose three or more times daily. The optimal frequency and timing of SMBG for patients with T2DM on oral agents are not known but should be sufficient to facilitate reaching glucose goals. Hb_{A1c} testing is recommended at least twice a year in patients who are meeting treatment goals and who have stable glycemic control, but it should be performed more frequently (quarterly) in those patients who are not meeting glycemic goals or whose therapy has been changed.[3] It should be kept in mind that the value of Hb_{A1c} testing is limited under conditions that affect erythrocyte turnover,[4] and hemoglobin variants must be considered, particularly when the Hb_{A1c} result does not correlate with the patient's clinical situation and SMBG readings.

Table 2.2 Components of diabetes self-management education
Diabetes overview
Nutrition plan
Exercise and activity recommendations
Indications and use of glucose monitoring devices
Review on prevention, detection, and treatment of acute and chronic diabetic complications • Foot, skin, and dental care • Signs and symptoms of hypoglycemia/hyperglycemia and appropriate treatment options • Sick-day guidelines
Management options for improving diabetes control • Oral antidiabetic agents • Insulin administration and devices
Smoking cessation
Review of preconception care, pregnancy, and gestational diabetes

In recent years, technologies for continuous monitoring of interstitial glucose, which correlates highly with blood glucose, have become available. The concentration of glucose is then measured with a glucose oxidase electrode detector. Some continuous glucose sensors have alarms for hypoglycemia and hyperglycemia. These systems require calibration with SMBG readings. Promising clinical studies have shown decreases in the mean time spent in hypoglycemic and hyperglycemic ranges compared with SMBG; however, long-term studies are needed to demonstrate improvements in long-term glucose control or reduction of diabetic complications.

Nephropathy screening and control

Diabetes is the most common cause of end-stage renal disease, accounting for one-third of all dialysis patients. Persistent microalbuminuria is the earliest clinical evidence of diabetic nephropathy. Analysis of a spot sample for the albumin-to-creatinine ratio is the best screening test. Accepted albumin-to-creatinine ratio values are normal, <30 μg/mg creatinine; microalbuminuria, 30 to 299 μg/mg creatinine; and clinical albuminuria, ≥300 μg/mg creatinine.[5] Subjects with T1DM should be screened after 5 years of disease duration and yearly thereafter. Patients with T2DM should be screened at diagnosis and yearly thereafter. Aggressive blood pressure control in diabetic patients with microalbuminuria using angiotensin-converting enzyme inhibitors (ACEIs) or angiotensin II receptor blockers (ARBs) has been shown to reduce proteinuria and to delay nephropathy progression.[6]

Serum creatinine should be measured annually for the estimation of glomerular filtration rate (GFR) in all adults with diabetes regardless of the degree of urinary albumin excretion. The serum creatinine level alone should be used not as a measure of kidney function but instead to calculate GFR and estimate the level of chronic kidney disease.[7] The Cockcroft-Gault equation is commonly used to estimate GFR:

$$[(140 - \text{Age [years]}) \times \text{Body Weight (kg)} \times k]/\text{Serum Creatinine (μmol/L)}$$

where k is a constant: 1.23 (males) or 1.04 (females). Normal range is >90 mL/min, and mild, moderate, and severe renal dysfunction are defined as a GFR of 60 to 90 mL/min, 30 to 60 mL/min, and 15 to 30 mL/min, respectively. Patients with end-stage renal disease have a GFR of <15 mL/min. Referral to a renal specialist should be considered when the estimated GFR has fallen below 30 to 60 mL/min or if difficulties occur in the management of hypertension or hyperkalemia.[8]

Retinopathy screening and control

Diabetic retinopathy is the most frequent cause of new cases of blindness among adults aged 20 to 74 years. Poor glycemic control and hypertension are established risk factors for the development of diabetic retinopathy.[9] Intensive diabetes management has been shown to prevent and/or delay the onset of diabetic retinopathy. Glaucoma, cataracts, and other disorders of the eye also occur earlier in people with diabetes and should also be evaluated. Early diagnosis and prompt application of laser photocoagulation surgery are useful in preventing vision loss. Screening recommendations in adults with T1DM include an initial dilated and comprehensive eye examination within 5 years of the diagnosis of diabetes. Adults with T2DM should have an initial dilated and comprehensive eye examination shortly following the diagnosis of diabetes. Subsequent examinations for patients with T1DM and T2DM should be repeated annually.[1] Examinations will be required more frequently if retinopathy is progressing or there is a change in or loss of vision.[9]

Neuropathy screening and control

The two most common types of diabetic neuropathy are distal symmetric polyneuropathy (DPN) and autonomic neuropathy. Improved glycemic control may prevent and slow progression but rarely reverses neuronal loss. Early recognition and appropriate management are important for treatment of symptoms and to identify subjects at higher risk of complications, including foot ulcers and lower extremity amputation.[10] Autonomic neuropathy can cause erectile dysfunction, constipation, gastroparesis, neurogenic bladder, brittle diabetes, and hypoglycemic autonomic failure.[11] Cardiovascular autonomic neuropathy is a recognized CVD risk factor characterized by resting tachycardia, postural hypotension, and increased cardiovascular morbidity and mortality. Patients with diabetes should be screened annually for peripheral neuropathy by pinprick sensation, vibration perception (using a 128 Hz tuning fork), 10 g monofilament pressure sensation at the distal plantar aspect of both great toes and metatarsal joints, and assessment of ankle reflexes.[1,10]

Cardiovascular disease risk reduction

Macrovascular disease (coronary artery disease, stroke, and peripheral vascular disease) is responsible for the majority of morbidity and mortality associated with diabetes.[12] Coronary artery disease is the leading cause of death among patients with T2DM, and women have a higher cardiovascular risk than do men. Adult subjects with T2DM, even if asymptomatic, are classified as having coronary heart disease equivalent and should be treated as if they have underlying CVD. Although observational and prospective studies have shown continuous associations of blood glucose and Hb_{A1c} levels with the risks of major vascular events,[13] randomized controlled trials evaluating the effects of tight glycemic control have failed to provide evidence that intensive glucose control reduces cardiovascular risk and mortality.[14–16] Two recently completed multicenter clinical trials, the ACCORD and the ADVANCE trials, reported that intensive therapy targeting an Hb_{A1c} below 6.0% and 6.5%, respectively, resulted in no significant reduction in major macrovascular events. In the ACCORD trial, deaths from any cause and from cardiovascular causes were significantly higher in the intensive therapy group than in the standard therapy group. It should be noted, however, that in the ACCORD trial the rate of nonfatal myocardial infarction was significantly lower in the intensive therapy group and that patients who did not have a history of a cardiovascular event or whose baseline Hb_{A1c} level was below 8% had significantly fewer fatal and nonfatal cardiovascular events. In addition, in the ADVANCE trial, intensive treatment resulted in a significant reduction in microvascular complications. The results of these recent studies indicate that a target Hb_{A1c} level of approximately 7% may be appropriate in this high-risk population and that it is clear that the prevention of macrovascular complications of diabetes requires a multifactorial approach addressing all major modifiable risk factors. The ADA and the American Heart Association have independently published guidelines for CVD prevention.[17] Extensive evidence from clinical trials indicates that in addition to targeting glycemic control, aggressive treatment of hypertension, dyslipidemia, and hypercoagulability prevents CVD events and can improve the event-free survival rate in people with diabetes who already have clinical CVD.[14,17] Screening recommendations and treatment goals are listed in Tables 2.3 and 2.4.

Blood pressure control

Hypertension affects more than half of patients with diabetes and represents a major risk factor for CVD and microvascular complications.

Table 2.3 Screening and preventive measures of microvascular complications

Complication	Screening method	Preventive measures
Nephropathy	Spot urine sample for albumin-to-creatinine ratio: • Normal: <30 μg/mg • Microalbuminuria: 30 to 299 μg/m • Albuminuria: ≥300 μ/mg Serum creatinine to estimate GFR Cockcroft-Gault equation: • Normal: >90 mL/min Renal dysfunction: • Mild: 60 to 90 mL/min • Moderate: 30 to 60 mL/min • Severe: 15 to 30 mL/min • End stage: <15 mL/min	T1DM screen within 5 years of diagnosis and yearly thereafter. T2DM screen at diagnosis and yearly thereafter. In addition to glycemic control, aggressive blood pressure control using ACE-I or ARBs reduces proteinuria and delays nephropathy progression.
Retinopathy	Dilated and comprehensive eye examination	T1DM screen within 5 years of diagnosis and yearly thereafter. T2DM screen at diagnosis and yearly thereafter. Intensive diabetes and blood pressure management prevent and delay the onset of retinopathy. Laser photocoagulation surgery is useful in preventing vision loss.
Neuropathy	Distal symmetric polyneuropathy (DPN): pinprick sensation (10 g monofilament), vibration perception (128 Hz tuning fork), and ankle reflexes. Autonomic neuropathy: history of erectile dysfunction, constipation, gastroparesis, neurogenic bladder, hypoglycemia unawareness, resting tachycardia, and postural hypotension.	Improved glycemic control may prevent and slow progression of diabetic neuropathy. Early recognition and management may relieve symptoms and prevent foot ulcers and lower extremity amputations. Cardiac autonomic neuropathy increases risk of cardiovascular morbidity and mortality.

Epidemiological and intervention studies have demonstrated a continuous relationship between the level of blood pressure and the risk of stroke, diabetes-related death, heart failure, and microvascular complications (UKPDS[14]). The primary goal of therapy for adults is to decrease blood pressure to <130/80 mmHg. Lifestyle modifications and a large number of pharmacological agents are available for controlling blood pressure in diabetic subjects.[1] Achieving the recommended blood pressure target,

Table 2.4 Preventing cardiovascular complications

Intervention	Screening method	Preventive measures
Blood pressure control	Check blood pressure at each visit. Target goal: <130/80 mmHg. Elevated values should be confirmed on a separate day.	Blood pressure control prevents microvascular and macrovascular complications. • Lifestyle modification (salt restriction, weight loss, increased physical activity) • Pharmacological intervention; multiple antihypertensive agents are frequently necessary
Lipid control	Low-risk adults (without CVD and under the age of 40): check lipid profile at initial visit and then every 2 years. Lipid targets: • LDL cholesterol <100 mg/dL • HDL cholesterol >50 mg/dL • Triglycerides <150 mg/dL For patients with known CVD check lipid profile at initial visit, then annually. Lipid targets: • LDL cholesterol <70 mg/dL • HDL cholesterol >50 mg/dL • Triglycerides <150 mg/dL	Statins are the drugs of choice for LDL reduction. Other drugs to be considered are nicotinic acid, ezetimibe, bile acid sequestrants, and fibric acid derivatives. Improve glycemic control in patients with high triglycerides and low HDL cholesterol. If necessary, use fibric acid derivatives or nicotinic acid. Combination therapy with a statin and a fibrate or statin and niacin may be used, but this combination is associated with an increased risk for abnormal transaminase levels and rhabdomyolysis.
Aspirin therapy	Aspirin therapy (75 to 162 mg/day) is indicated as a primary prevention strategy in subjects with T1DM and T2DM >40 years of age, family history of CVD, hypertension, smoking, dyslipidemia, or albuminuria. Aspirin therapy (75 to 162 mg/day) as a secondary prevention strategy is indicated in subjects with T1DM and T2DM with a history of CVD.	Aspirin therapy lowers by about one-fourth the risk of myocardial infarction, stroke, and transient ischemic attacks. In people with aspirin allergy, bleeding tendency, or with recent gastrointestinal bleeding the use of clopidogrel is an alternative to aspirin therapy. Aspirin is not recommended for CVD prevention in people <30 years of age.
Smoking cessation	All subjects with diabetes should receive appropriate smoking cessation counseling.	Smoking is associated with increased risk of CVD, microvascular complications, and premature death. All subjects should be advised not to smoke.

however, is not easy, and more than half of hypertensive patients with diabetes are not at the goal. Many patients will require three or more drugs to reach target goals.[18] Weight loss, increased physical activity, smoking cessation, and reduction of sodium and alcohol intake are associated with substantial improvements in blood pressure. Antihypertensive agents, including angiotensin-converting enzyme inhibitors (ACEIs), angiotensin II receptor blockers (ARBs), β-blockers, diuretics, and calcium channel blockers, have been shown to be effective in reducing cardiovascular events. ACEIs and ARBs have been shown to prevent the development and progression of nephropathy as well as reduce major CVD outcomes.[18]

Lipid control

Diabetic dyslipidemia is characterized by multiple lipoprotein defects, including moderate-high levels of total and LDL cholesterol, triglycerides, and small dense LDL particles and low levels of HDL cholesterol. Patients with diabetes have a three-fold higher mortality rate for cardiovascular events at each level of serum cholesterol compared with the nondiabetic population. The primary target for patients with diabetes is an LDL cholesterol level of <100 mg/dL.[1] A tighter target (<70 mg/dL) may be appropriate in patients at high risk or with known CVD. In the U.K. Prospective Diabetes Study, a 1.57-fold increased risk of coronary heart disease was reported for every 1 mmol/L increment in LDL cholesterol.[14] In the Heart Protection Study,[19] 5963 U.K. adults (aged 40 to 80 years) known to have diabetes and an additional 14,573 adults with occlusive arterial disease (but without diagnosed diabetes) were randomly allocated to receive 40 mg simvastatin daily or placebo. With an average difference in LDL cholesterol of 1.0 mmol/L (39 mg/dL) during the 5-year treatment period, both diabetic and nondiabetic subjects experienced a highly significant reduction of about 25% in the first event rate for major coronary events, for strokes, and for revascularizations. Among diabetic patients, 5 years of statin treatment prevented about 45 people per 1000 from having at least one major vascular event.[19]

Statins are the drugs of choice for LDL reduction.[20] Other drugs that lower LDL include nicotinic acid, ezetimibe, bile acid sequestrants, and fibric acid derivatives. High triglycerides resulting from an increased production of triglyceride-rich lipoproteins and impaired clearance of VLDL is the most common dyslipidemia in diabetes. Some patients with high triglycerides may be more responsive to improvement of glycemic control and may achieve desirable levels even without lipid-lowering drugs. If these measures are not sufficient, fibric acid derivatives or nicotinic acid can be used to control hypertriglyceridemia. Combination therapy, with a statin and a fibrate or a statin and niacin, may be efficacious for treatment for all three lipid fractions, but this combination is associated with an increased risk for abnormal transaminase levels, myositis, or rhabdomyolysis. The risk of rhabdomyolysis is higher with higher doses of statins and with renal insufficiency and seems to be lower when statins are combined with fenofibrate than gemfibrozil.

Aspirin therapy

Aspirin therapy (75 to 162 mg/day) is recommended for primary prevention of cardiovascular events in subjects with T1DM and T2DM over

30 years of age, a family history of CVD, hypertension, smoking, dyslipidemia, or albuminuria. Aspirin therapy (75 to 325 mg/day) is recommended for secondary prevention in subjects with a history of CVD or hypertension. Several clinical trials have shown a greater than 30% decrease in myocardial infarction and a 20% decrease in stroke in patients with a history of CVD.[21] Aspirin therapy is not recommended for patients under the age of 30 due to lack of evidence of benefit and is contraindicated in patients under the age of 20 years because of the associated risk of Reye's syndrome. In people with aspirin allergy, bleeding tendency, or recent gastrointestinal bleeding, the use of clopidogrel may be a reasonable alternative to aspirin therapy.[22]

Smoking cessation

Smoking is associated with an increased risk of CVD, microvascular complications, and premature death in subjects with T1DM and T2DM. A number of large randomized clinical trials have demonstrated the efficacy and cost-effectiveness of smoking cessation counseling in changing smoking behavior and reducing tobacco use. Thus all subjects with diabetes should receive appropriate smoking cessation counseling. Special considerations should include assessment of level of nicotine dependence, which is associated with difficulty in quitting and relapse.[1]

Summary of practice guidelines for health care professionals should be readily accessible on patient charts, in examining rooms, or on office electronic tracking systems. The use of checklists or automatic reminders to health care professionals may prompt providers to adhere to guidelines. A variety of paper-form tracking systems (Table 2.5) and computerized systems may increase adherence and can help in improving care to subjects with diabetes.

Table 2.5 Office flow sheet for diabetes care				
Name: **D.O.B.:**	**Date**	**Date**	**Date**	**Date**
Weight				
Blood pressure				
Foot exam √ when done				
Review blood glucose records √ when done				
Exercise counseling √ when done				
Dietary counseling √ when done				
Smoking cessation counseling √ when done				
Psychosocial assessment √ when done				
Dilated eye exam √ when done				
Flu shot √ when done				
Hb_{A1c}				
LDL cholesterol				
HDL cholesterol				
Triglycerides				

References

1. Standards of medical care in diabetes—2008. *Diabetes Care.* 2008;31(suppl 1): S12–S54.

2. Norris SL, Lau J, Smith SJ, Schmid CH, Engelgau MM. Self-management education for adults with type 2 diabetes: a meta-analysis of the effect on glycemic control. *Diabetes Care.* 2002;25:1159–1171.

3. Welschen LM, Bloemendal E, Nijpels G, et al. Self-monitoring of blood glucose in patients with type 2 diabetes who are not using insulin: a systematic review. *Diabetes Care.* 2005;28:1510–1517.

4. Smiley D, Dagogo-Jack S, Umpierrez G. Therapy insight: metabolic and endocrine disorders in sickle cell disease. *Nat Clin Pract Endocrinol Metab.* 2008;4:102–109.

5. Garg JP, Bakris GL. Microalbuminuria: marker of vascular dysfunction, risk factor for cardiovascular disease. *Vasc Med.* 2002;7:35–43.

6. Bakris GL, Williams M, Dworkin L, et al. Preserving renal function in adults with hypertension and diabetes: a consensus approach. National Kidney Foundation Hypertension and Diabetes Executive Committees Working Group. *Am J Kidney Dis.* 2000;36:646–661.

7. Bailie GR, Uhlig K, Levey AS. Clinical practice guidelines in nephrology: evaluation, classification, and stratification of chronic kidney disease. *Pharmacotherapy.* 2005;25:491–502.

8. Rigalleau V, Lasseur C, Perlemoine C, et al. Estimation of glomerular filtration rate in diabetic subjects: Cockcroft formula or modification of Diet in Renal Disease study equation? *Diabetes Care.* 2005;28:838–843.

9. Ciulla TA, Amador AG, Zinman B. Diabetic retinopathy and diabetic macular edema: pathophysiology, screening, and novel therapies. *Diabetes Care.* 2003;26:2653–2664.

10. Boulton AJ, Vinik AI, Arezzo JC, et al. Diabetic neuropathies: a statement by the American Diabetes Association. *Diabetes Care.* 2005;28:956–962.

11. Vinik AI, Maser RE, Mitchell BD, Freeman R. Diabetic autonomic neuropathy. *Diabetes Care.* 2003;26:1553–1579.

12. Fox CS, Coady S, Sorlie PD, et al. Increasing cardiovascular disease burden due to diabetes mellitus: the Framingham Heart Study. *Circulation.* 2007;115:1544–1550.

13. Selvin E, Marinopoulos S, Berkenblit G, et al. Meta-analysis: glycosylated hemoglobin and cardiovascular disease in diabetes mellitus. *Ann Intern Med.* 2004;141:421–431.

14. U.K. Prospective Diabetes Study 16. Overview of 6 years' therapy of type II diabetes: a progressive disease. U.K. Prospective Diabetes Study Group. *Diabetes.* 1995;44:1249–1258.

15. Gerstein HC, Miller ME, Byington RP, et al. Effects of intensive glucose lowering in type 2 diabetes. *N Engl J Med.* 2008;358:2545–2559.

16. Patel A, MacMahon S, Chalmers J, et al. Intensive blood glucose control and vascular outcomes in patients with type 2 diabetes. *N Engl J Med.* 2008;358:2560–2572.

17. Buse JB, Ginsberg HN, Bakris GL, et al. Primary prevention of cardiovascular diseases in people with diabetes mellitus: a scientific statement from the American Heart Association and the American Diabetes Association. *Circulation.* 2007;115:114–126.

18. Arauz-Pacheco C, Parrott MA, Raskin P. The treatment of hypertension in adult patients with diabetes. *Diabetes Care.* 2002;25:134–147.

19. Collins R, Armitage J, Parish S, Sleigh P, Peto R. MRC/BHF Heart Protection Study of cholesterol-lowering with simvastatin in 5963 people with diabetes: a randomised placebo-controlled trial. *Lancet.* 2003;361:2005–2016.

20. Haffner SM. Dyslipidemia management in adults with diabetes. *Diabetes Care.* 2004;27(suppl 1):S68–S71.

21. Baigent C, Sudlow C, Collius R, Peto R, and the Antithrombotic Trialists' Collaboration. Collaborative meta-analysis of randomised trials of antiplatelet therapy for prevention of death, myocardial infarction, and stroke in high risk patients. *BMJ.* 2002;324:71–86.

22. Wackers FJ, Young LH, Inzucchi SE, et al. Detection of silent myocardial ischemia in asymptomatic diabetic subjects: the DIAD study. *Diabetes Care.* 2004;27:1954–1961.

Chapter 3

Pharmacological treatment of type 2 diabetes

Vivian Fonseca

Although insulin is very effective in the treatment of type 2 diabetes mellitus (T2DM), most patients and physicians prefer to use other agents first. We will therefore consider first the noninsulin agents in the treatment of diabetes. As the disease progresses, many, if not all, of these agents will likely have to be used in combination with insulin. The American Diabetes Association (ADA) and European Association for the Study of Diabetes (EASD) consensus statement recommended a treatment algorithm promoting preferential use of older, less expensive agents, including metformin, sulfonylureas, and insulin (Fig. 3.1), in treating patients, but it leaves room for the flexibility that is necessary in clinical practice to individualize treatments and goals.[1]

Treatment decisions are typically individualized based on multiple factors that may be weighted differently in the guidelines than in clinical practice. Physicians make treatment decisions based on their clinical assessments of their patients' health and comorbid conditions, treatment adherence, tendency to experience side effects, motivation to improve and/or avoid insulin, and many other factors. Decisions also may be influenced by formulary restrictions, as well as costs. Because insulin treatment is discussed in a separate chapter, we review only other agents here.

Lifestyle changes

Lifestyle change should be the cornerstone of diabetes management. The term includes increased physical activity and, when appropriate, a change in diet to decrease glycemic excursions and induce weight loss. A detailed discussion of strategies to change lifestyle can be found in other chapters. However, it is important in the context of this chapter to state that without lifestyle change, it is challenging to manage T2DM. Higher doses of medications need to be used, and weight gain as a side effect of medication becomes a major problem.

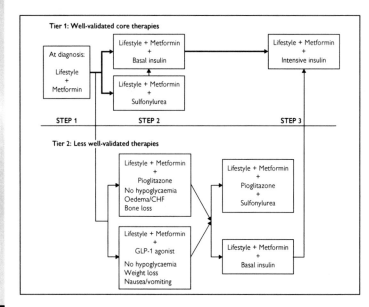

Figure 3.1 Updated algorithm for the metabolic management of type 2 diabetes.

Pharmacological therapy

Eight different classes of medication, in addition to insulin, are currently approved for treatment of hyperglycemia in T2DM. Beneficial effects of antihyperglycemic agents appear to be mediated predominantly through their ability to lower blood glucose. Studies are currently in progress to determine whether any particular agent (or treatment strategy) has specific advantages, beyond glucose lowering, in terms of reducing cardiovascular end points.[2]

Unfortunately, there are few high-quality head-to-head comparison trials evaluating the ability of available noninsulin agents to achieve recommended glycemic targets. This is important because the glucose-lowering effectiveness of individual medications is strongly influenced by baseline characteristics such as Hb_{A1c} level, duration of diabetes, and previous therapy. Although some publications make comparisons of the relative glucose-lowering effectiveness of available agents based on their package insert data, such comparisons are problematic. A few comparative trials demonstrate that the effects of most agents on glucose is similar across and within drug classes and the glucose-lowering capability is most closely related with the baseline Hb_{A1c}.[3]

No single treatment strategy has been shown to be superior for all patients. Decisions about which medication or combination of medications to use should be made based on their effects on Hb_{A1c} levels, contraindications, side-effect profiles, patient preferences, and costs.

Table 3.1 outlines the mechanism of action, dosing characteristics, contraindications, side effects, and costs of available noninsulin therapies. Each class of medications is briefly discussed next.

Metformin

Metformin, the only biguanide available, works primarily by decreasing hepatic glucose production and has the advantages of not causing hypoglycemia and being associated with weight loss. In the U.K. Prospective Diabetes Study (UKPDS), metformin was shown to have a beneficial effect on CVD outcomes.[4] Although treatment failure in the UKPDS was high, in the ADOPT study,[5] glycemic control with metformin was significantly better maintained compared with use of a sulfonylurea. Because of these results, metformin has been recommended by the ADA/EASD not only as the first-line treatment of choice but also to be started at the time of diagnosis of T2DM.

Metformin has also been extensively tested in combination with all the other treatments, including insulin, and has been shown to have a beneficial effect in combination. Most important, it may attenuate the weight gain cause by other agents, including insulin.

The most common adverse effects are diarrhea and nausea. Lactic acidosis, a potentially fatal adverse effect, is extremely rare and is associated almost exclusively with other risk factors such as renal or hepatic disease.

We have attempted to modify the approach recommended by the ADA/EASD algorithm to demonstrate possible pathways for patients to reach their goal with metformin-based therapy, unless it is not tolerated or contraindicated (Fig. 3.2).

Sulfonylureas

Sulfonylureas reduce blood glucose levels by stimulating insulin secretion by the pancreatic β cells. The combination of their proven efficacy, low incidence of adverse events, and low cost has contributed to their success and continued use. They are particularly effective in the treatment of symptomatic patients because of their quick onset of action and because, at least in the short term, they are very effective.

Sulfonylureas have been shown to be particularly effective in specific inherited forms of diabetes. For example, neonatal diabetes due to a mutation in the Kir channel (which actually also serves as the sulfonylurea receptor) is particularly responsive to this class of drugs. Similar superior efficacy has been demonstrated compared with metformin in patients with mutations causing maturity-onset diabetes of the young (MODY).

The major adverse side effect of sulfonylureas is hypoglycemia, which appears to occur most frequently in the elderly. Fortunately, severe episodes tend to be rare. Hypoglycemia may be less common with glimepiride compared with glyburide, possibly due to a shorter half-life and differences in receptor binding characteristics. A weight gain of about 2 kg is common with sulfonylurea therapy. The major problem with sulfonylureas is their inability to change the natural history of the disease and continued loss of β-cell function over time, rendering them ineffective.[5] They also

Table 3.1 Mechanisms of action and prescribing considerations of diabetes treatments

Class	Site of action	Mechanism of action	Contraindications	Advantages	Disadvantages
Biguanides	Liver	Decrease glucose production	Creatinine >1.5 man, >1.4 woman CHF requiring treatment Acute illness	No weight gain Decreased mortality and CV events	Diarrhea
Sulfonylureas	Pancreas	Increase insulin secretion		Inexpensive	Hypoglycemia
Meglitinides	Pancreas	Increase insulin secretion		Short-acting	
Thiazolidinediones	Muscle, fat	Increase glucose uptake	ALT > 2.5 ×ULN CHF	Treat insulin resistance	Edema, CHF
α-glucosidase inhibitors	Gut	Delay carbohydrate absorption	Chronic intestinal disorders Cirrhosis Serum creatinine >2.0 mg/dL	Nonsystemic, target postprandial glucose	Flatulence
DPP-4 inhibitors	Pancreas	Prolongs effect of GLP-1 (↑ insulin, ↓ glucagon)	None	Well tolerated	Expensive, very little long-term data
GLP-1 analogues	Pancreas, stomach ? Brain	Similar effects as GLP-1 (↑ insulin, ↓ glucagon, ↑ satiety, delayed gastric emptying)	Severe renal insufficiency (CrCl < 30 mL/min)	Weight loss	Nausea Very little long-term data
Amylin analogues	Pancreas, stomach	Decreased nutrient delivery to jejunum,↓ glucagon, ↑ satiety, delays gastric emptying	Gastroparesis	Weight loss	Nausea, injections, Risk of hypoglycemia if food is absorbed too late and insulin is working
Bile acid Sequestrants (Colesevelam)	Gut	Unclear	GI problems	Non systemic lowers LDL	Modest effect; raised Tg
Dopamine Agonists (Bromocriptine)	Brain	Unclear (insulin sensitizer)	None	Novel mechanism	Nausea/ vomiting

ALT, alanine transaminase; CHF, congestive heart failure; CrCl, creatinine clearance; NYHA, New York Heart Association.

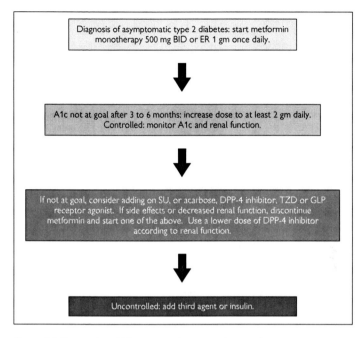

Figure 3.2 Proposed model for using metformin to achieve goal.

have no effect on cardiovascular function and indeed have some theoretical disadvantages. The package inserts of sulfonylureas include a warning of increased cardiovascular risk. However, no such increased risk was seen in the UKPDS.[6]

Other secretagogues (meglitinides)

Two agents—repaglinide and nateglinide—are available in the meglitinides class. Like sulfonylureas, they stimulate insulin secretion by binding to the sulfonylurea receptor. They have a more rapid onset and shorter duration of action than the sulfonylureas and are designed to target postprandial hyperglycemia. They should be taken just prior to meals. Compared with sulfonylureas, the risk for hypoglycemia is similar with repaglinide but less frequent with nateglinide.[7] There are insufficient data on the long-term effects of these drugs. Since they bind to the sulfonylurea receptor, one has to assume there are similar long-term effects to those in that class.

Thiazolidinediones

Two thiazolidinediones (glitazones or TZDs)—rosiglitazone and pioglitazone—are currently available. Their main mechanism of action relates to their binding to and serving as an agonist to a transcription factor called peroxisome proliferator activator receptor gamma (PPAR γ). This results in changes to the transcription of several genes involved in insulin action and glucose metabolism—improving insulin sensitivity. They lower blood glucose primarily by increasing insulin-mediated glucose uptake in muscle and adipocytes. To a lesser extent, they decrease hepatic glucose production. Like metformin, TZDs do not cause hypoglycemia when used as monotherapy or in combination with other agents that also do not cause hypoglycemia. Thus, a combination of metformin and a TZD is attractive in that it will not cause hypoglycemia and will improve insulin sensitivity in different organs. A significant advantage of the TZDs is that they have been shown to have the lowest rate of pancreatic failure alone or in combination.[5,8] They have been extensively tested as monotherapy as well as in combination with other agents, including insulin.

The major side effects of TZDs are weight gain and fluid retention. The fluid retention typically manifests as peripheral edema, although new or worsened congestive heart failure can occur. There has been some controversy about the effect of TZDs on cardiovascular risk.[9–11] Clinical trial data suggest that pioglitazone may have cardiovascular benefits.[11,12] Pioglitazone decreases plasma triglycerides, an effect which was not seen with rosiglitazone in a trial comparing the two drugs. However, both agents raise HDL cholesterol, and while they increase LDL cholesterol, the LDL particle size increases (making it less atherogenic), and this effect may be countered by concomitant statin use. Studies that are currently in progress will further help to determine the effects of TZDs on CVD risk.[2,12] Furthermore, both rosiglitazone and pioglitazone may increase the risk of fracture, a complication that already is increased in patients with diabetes. These agents should be avoided in patients with congestive heart failure and those with an increased risk for fracture and used cautiously in those treated with insulin. Indeed the package insert for rosiglitazone states that it is not recommended in patients treated with insulin and also those treated with nitrates. On the other hand such patients were included in the PROACTIVE trial with pioglitazone, without adverse outcomes.

α-glucosidase inhibitors

Acarbose and miglitol are the two agents in the α-glucosidase inhibitor (AGI) class of diabetes medications. They reduce the rate of digestion of polysaccharides in the proximal small intestine. When used before meals, they delay the absorption of complex carbohydrates and blunt postprandial hyperglycemia, resulting in modest reductions in Hb_{A1c}. They are not associated with weight changes or hypoglycemia. The main limitations to their widespread use are the need for frequent dosing and poor tolerability due to frequent gastrointestinal side effects. On the other hand, they have been shown to be effective in patients with impaired glucose tolerance, not only decreasing the progression to diabetes but also decreasing cardiovascular events.[13,14]

Colesevelam

Bile acid sequestrants have long been approved for the lowering of plasma cholesterol. There have been suggestions that they may also lower glucose. This has now been convincingly demonstrated in several clinical trials with colesevelam, which has now been approved for the treatment of diabetes.[15,16] While the glucose lowering effect appears to be relatively small, it comes in addition to the effect on lipids, thus providing a reduction in 2 factors. Furthermore, the drug is not absorbed and does not have serious systemic side effects, through constipation may be a limiting factor.

Bromocriptine

A quick release form of Bromocriptine (a drug long used in the treatment of pituitary disorders) has been approved for the treatment of type 2 diabetes. It increases brain dopamine levels and in doing so exerts an insulin sensitizing effect. In clinical trials it has a modest effect on glucose control in combination with many other therapies. It should be started in a dose of 0.8 mg once daily orally, and gradually increased to 4.8mg. It should only be given in the mornings. Side effects include nausea and vomiting and dizziness.

GLP-1 analogues

Exenatide and liraglutide are members of this new class of agents, the GLP-1 analogues. Because they resist degradation by dipeptidyl peptidase IV (DPP-IV), they have significantly longer half-lives than natural GLP-1, but they exhibit many of the same properties of GLP-1. They enhance "glucose-dependent" insulin secretion (importantly, they do not stimulate such secretion during hypoglycemia), suppress hepatic glucagon secretion, slow gastric emptying, and reduce food intake.

Although only modest improvements in glycemic control have been demonstrated with exenatide,[17,18] it does not cause hypoglycemia and is associated with moderate weight loss, which makes it a very attractive choice for obese patients with diabetes who are trying to lose weight. Exenatide is usually used in combination with a range of oral agents. For patients failing on oral agents, it is a potential alternative to insulin therapy, with the advantage of weight loss rather than weight gain.[19]

The major limitations to the widespread use of exanatide are the relatively high frequency of gastrointestinal side effects and the

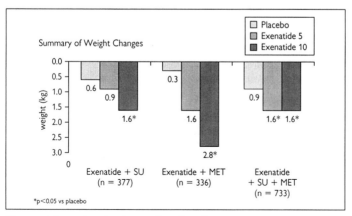

Figure 3.3 Exenatide and oral agents. The effect of exenatide on body weight in 3 pivotal trials.[20–22] Adapted from Buse JB et al. *Diabetes Care.* 2004;27:2628–2635; Defronzo RA et al., *Diabetes Care.* 2005;28:1092–1100; Kendall DM et al. *Diabetes Care.* 2005;28:1083–1091.

requirement for twice-daily injections. A few cases of pancreatitis with exanatide treatment have been reported, but this complication is relatively uncommon. Similar new agents in this class, including a preparation that will require only a single weekly injection, are currently being evaluated in clinical trials. No long-term studies are available with exenatide (Figure 3.3).

Liraglutide has 97% amino acid sequence homology with endogenous human GLP-1(7-37). Resistance to metabolic degradation by both DPP-IV and neutral endopeptidase (NEP) gives liraglutide a plasma half-life of 13 hours and makes it suitable for once daily injection. Serious hypoglycemia can occur when liraglutide is used with an insulin secretagogue such as sulfonylurea; risk may be reduced by lowering the dose of the insulin secretagogue. There are no conclusive data establishing a risk of pancreatitis for liraglutide treatment; patients taking the agent should be observed carefully and the agent discontinued promptly if pancreatitis is suspected. The most commonly reported gastrointestinal side effects are nausea and diarrhea.

Dipeptidyl peptidase IV (DPP-IV) inhibitors

Dipeptidyl peptidase IV (DPP-IV) inhibitors are a relatively new class of drugs for the treatment of type 2 diabetes. Sitagliptin was the first agent in this class to be approved in the United States, followed recently by Saxagliptin. Another agent, vildagliptin, is undergoing U.S. Food and Drug Administration review, and is marketed in several other countries. Several other drugs in this class are in development. By inhibiting the enzyme DPP-IV, the enzyme that normally inactivates GLP-1, these agents prolong the glucoregulatory actions of GLP-1.[18,19] DPP-IV inhibitors modestly reduce HbA1c levels, are generally very well tolerated, are not associated with hypoglycemia, and are weight neutral. Their good tolerability and ease of use makes them an attractive option for patient in primary care as well as in elderly patients. Some skin rashes, including Stevens-Johnson syndrome, have been occasionally reported in patients treated with sitagliptin, and the long-term effects of these agents remain unknown. Since sitagliptin is excreted by the kidney and accumulates in the body in renal failure, the dose should be reduced by 50–75% in patient with moderate and severe renal impairment respectively. Other agents in the class that are not excreted by the kidney may not need such dose adjustment (Figure 3.4).

Amylin mimetics

Pramlintide is a synthetic analogue of amylin, a hormone that is synthesized by pancreatic β cells and co-secreted with insulin in response to a meal. Treatment, which requires injections before each meal, is associated with mild reductions in A1C and weight loss.[22] Treatment with pramlintide thus represents a physiological replacement therapy for both type 1 and type 2 diabetes but is approved only in combination with prandial insulin injections. On the other hand, this may be a disadvantage as it cannot be mixed with insulin and therefore requires multiple injections. However, for patients taking insulin, it offers the potential for weight loss, as well as decreasing postprandial fluctuations in glucose while taking less insu-

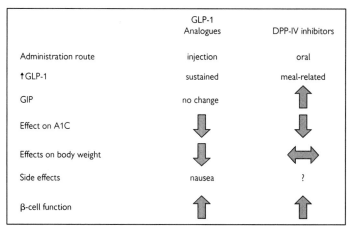

	GLP-1 Analogues	DPP-IV inhibitors
Administration route	injection	oral
↑GLP-1	sustained	meal-related
GIP	no change	⬆
Effect on A1C	⬇	⬇
Effects on body weight	⬇	⬌
Side effects	nausea	?
β-cell function	⬆	⬆

Figure 3.4 Comparison of the two classes of drugs affecting the incretin system—GLP-1 agonists and DPP-IV inhibitors.

lin. It decreases stomach emptying and suppresses postprandial glucagon secretion. Nausea is a common side effect.

Approaches to the treatment of patients

The treatment paradigm has changed considerably over the past few years. Following data from the UKPDS demonstrating the value of metformin as first-line therapy for T2DM, several organizations have recommended that metformin therapy be initiated at the time of diagnosis. However, a goal-oriented approach should be taken and additional therapy instituted rapidly should the patient fail to achieve goals or, after achieving the glycemic goal, the blood sugar level rises and further therapy becomes necessary, as summarized in Figures 3.1 and 3.2. Early institution of treatment for diabetes, at a time when the Hb_{A1c} is not significantly elevated, has been associated with improved glycemic control over time and decreased long-term complications.[23]

Initial treatment for most patients is a single oral agent, although insulin may be preferred if the patient has very high initial blood glucose levels, is underweight, is losing weight, or is ketotic.

Combination therapy

Even if oral-agent monotherapy is initially effective, glycemic control is likely to deteriorate over time due to progressive loss of β-cell function in T2DM. Although metformin is generally recommended as first-line therapy, there is no consensus as to what the second-line agent should be, and this selection is likely to remain controversial until clinical trials comparing various combinations of drugs are carried out.[12] Numerous two-drug combinations have been studied and have been found to be effective.[18,24,25]

Selection of a second agent, from a different class from the first agent, should be made based on potential advantages and disadvantages. Potential advantages affecting choice of therapy include ease of use, synergistic effects (e.g., metformin and DPP-IV inhibition), targeting insulin resistance in different ways (metformin and TZDs), or lower cost (metformin and sulfonylureas). On the other hand, disadvantages may include a potential for increased side effects (metformin and sulfonylurea[26]) or high cost if two relatively new and expensive drugs are used in combination.

If patients progress to the point where dual therapy does not provide adequate control, either a third noninsulin agent or insulin can be added. In an interesting study mentioned earlier, such patients were randomized to exenatide or insulin. Both agents reduced Hb_{A1c} significantly, but insulin treatment led to weight gain and exenatide treatment led to weight loss over 6 months.[19] The long-term management of such patients, however, is unclear, and only insulin therapy has been studied long term and is clearly safe and effective. Combination of insulin with metformin may attenuate weight gain and also improve glycemic control. Considerations at this point include costs, complexity of treatment, and level of Hb_{A1c}. Patients with significantly elevated Hb_{A1c} levels on two noninsulin agents are more likely to achieve goals with insulin. While insulin treatment is discussed elsewhere, it is important to recognize that many of the treatments discussed here can be combined with insulin (except for the incretin mimetics and enhancers, which have not been well studied with insulin).

New guidelines

Recently the ADA/EASD updated its consensus statement on medical management of hyperglycemia.[27] The algorithm in figure 3.1 has been updated to reflect concerns about the TZDs (which are now considered tier 2 drugs), the availability of GPL-1 agonists, as well as other new agents and the newest consensus of the ADA/EASD. It is important to also recognize that there is an emphasis on individualization of goals and strategies to get to those goals. By their very nature, consensus statements are based on varying levels of evidence and are always subject to change when new evidence becomes available.

Conclusions

Over the past decade, there have been enormous advances in the understanding of T2DM and its complications. This has resulted in the development of multiple new glucose-lowering medications, which can be used alone or in combinations. Multiple combinations can be used effectively. The combination of these agents with insulin is also possible. In order for patients to achieve glucose goals, treatment must be promptly initiated, carefully monitored, and rapidly advanced.

References

1. Nathan DM, Buse JB, Davidson MB, et al. Management of hyperglycemia in type 2 diabetes: a consensus algorithm for the initiation and adjustment of therapy: update regarding thiazolidinediones: a consensus statement from the American Diabetes Association and the European Association for the Study of Diabetes. *Diabetes Care.* 2008;31:173–175.

2. Magee MF, Isley WL, BARI 2D Trial Investigators. Rationale, design, and methods for glycemic control in the Bypass Angioplasty Revascularization Investigation 2 Diabetes (BARI 2D) trial. *Am J Cardiol.* 2006;97:20G–30G.

3. Bloomgarden ZT, Dodis R, Viscoli CM, Holmboe ES, Inzucchi SE. Lower baseline glycemia reduces apparent oral agent glucose-lowering efficacy: a meta-regression analysis. *Diabetes Care.* 2006;29:2137–2139.

4. UK Prospective Diabetes Study (UKPDS) Group. Effect of intensive blood-glucose control with metformin on complications in overweight patients with type 2 diabetes (UKPDS 34). *Lancet.* 1998;352:854–865.

5. Kahn SE, Haffner SM, Heise MA, et al. Glycemic durability of rosiglitazone, metformin, or glyburide monotherapy. *N Engl J Med.* 2006;355:2427–2443.

6. UK Prospective Diabetes Study (UKPDS) Group. Intensive blood-glucose control with sulphonylureas or insulin compared with conventional treatment and risk of complications in patients with type 2 diabetes (UKPDS 33). *Lancet.* 1998;352:837–853.

7. Fonseca VA, Kelley DE, Cefalu W, et al. Hypoglycemic potential of nateglinide versus glyburide in patients with type 2 diabetes mellitus. *Metab Clin Exp.* 2004;53:1331–1335.

8. Matthews DR, Charbonnel BH, Hanefeld M, Brunetti P, Schernthaner G. Long-term therapy with addition of pioglitazone to metformin compared with the addition of gliclazide to metformin in patients with type 2 diabetes: a randomized, comparative study. *Diabetes Metab Res Rev.* 2005;21:167–174.

9. Nissen SE, Wolski K. Effect of rosiglitazone on the risk of myocardial infarction and death from cardiovascular causes. *N Engl J Med.* 2007;356:2457–2471.

10. Fonseca V, Jawa A, Asnani S. Commentary: the PROactive study—the glass is half full. *J Clin Endocrinol Metab.* 2006;91:25–27.

11. Dormandy JA, Charbonnel B, Eckland DJ, et al. Secondary prevention of macrovascular events in patients with type 2 diabetes in the PROactive study (PROspective pioglitAzone clinical trial in macroVascular events): a randomised controlled trial. *Lancet.* 2005;366:1279–1289.

12. Home PD, Pocock SJ, Beck-Nielsen H, et al. Rosiglitazone evaluated for cardiovascular outcomes—an interim analysis. *N Engl J Med.* 2007;357:28–38.

13. Chiasson JL, Josse RG, Gomis R, Hanefeld M, Karasik A, Laakso M. Acarbose treatment and the risk of cardiovascular disease and hypertension in patients with impaired glucose tolerance: the STOP-NIDDM trial. *JAMA.* 2003;290:486–494.

14. Hanefeld M, Chiasson JL, Koehler C, Henkel E, Schaper F, Temelkova-Kurktschiev T. Acarbose slows progression of intima-media thickness of the carotid arteries in subjects with impaired glucose tolerance. *Stroke.* 2004;35:1073–1078.

15. Goldberg RB, Fonseca VA, Truitt KE, Jones MR. Efficacy and safety of Colesevelam in patients with type 2 diabetes mellitus and inadequate glycemic control receiving insulin-based therapy. *Arch Intern Med.* 2008;168:1531–1540.

16. Fonseca VA, Rosenstock J, Wang AC, Truitt KE, Jones MR, Colesevelam HCl improves glycemic control and reduces LDL cholesterol in patients with inadequately controlled type 2 diabetes on sulfonylurea-based therapy. *Diabetes Care.* 2008;31:1479–1484.

17. Amori RE, Lau J, Pittas AG. Efficacy and safety of incretin therapy in type 2 diabetes: systematic review and meta-analysis. *JAMA.* 2007;298:194–206.

18. DeFronzo RA, Ratner RE, Han J, Kim DD, Fineman MS, Baron AD. Effects of exenatide (Exendin-4) on glycemic control and weight over 30 weeks in metformin-treated patients with type 2 diabetes. *Diabetes Care.* 2005;28:1092–1100.

19. Heine RJ, Van Gaal LF, Johns D, et al. Exenatide versus insulin glargine in patients with suboptimally controlled type 2 diabetes: a randomized trial. *Ann Intern Med.* 2005;143:559–569.

20. Amori RE, Lau J, Pittas AG. Efficacy and safety of incretin therapy in type 2 diabetes: systematic review and meta-analysis. *JAMA.* 2007;298:194–206.

21. Ahren B. Dipeptidyl peptidase-4 inhibitors: clinical data and clinical implications. *Diabetes Care.* 2007;30:1344–1350.

22. Hollander PA, Levy P, Fineman MS, et al. Pramlintide as an adjunct to insulin therapy improves long-term glycemic and weight control in patients with type 2 diabetes: a 1-year randomized controlled trial. *Diabetes Care.* 2003;26:784–790.

23. Colagiuri S, Cull CA, Holman RR, UKPDS Group. Are lower fasting plasma glucose levels at diagnosis of type 2 diabetes associated with improved outcomes? U.K. Prospective Diabetes Study 61. *Diabetes Care.* 2002;25:1410–1417.

24. Fonseca V, Rosenstock J, Patwardhan R, Salzman A. Effect of metformin and rosiglitazone combination therapy in patients with type 2 diabetes mellitus: a randomized controlled trial. *JAMA.* 2000;283:1695–1702.

25. Charbonnel B, Karasik A, Liu J, Wu M, Meininger G; Sitagliptin Study 020 Group. Efficacy and safety of the dipeptidyl peptidase-4 inhibitor sitagliptin added to ongoing metformin therapy in patients with type 2 diabetes inadequately controlled with metformin alone. *Diabetes Care.* 2006;29:2638–2643.

26. Turner RC, Cull CA, Frighi V, Holman RR. Glycemic control with diet, sulfonylurea, metformin, or insulin in patients with type 2 diabetes mellitus: progressive requirement for multiple therapies (UKPDS 49). UK Prospective Diabetes Study (UKPDS) Group. *JAMA.* 1999;281:2005–2012.

27. Nathan DM, Buse JB, Davidson MB, Ferrannini E, Holman RR, Sherwin R, Zinman B. Management of hyperglycemia in type 2 diabetes: a consensus algorithm for the initiation and adjustment of therapy: update regarding thiazolidinediones: a consensus statement from the American Diabetes Association and the European Association for the Study of Diabetes. *Diabetes Care.* 2009; 32(1):193–203.

Chapter 4

Insulin therapy in ambulatory patients with type 2 diabetes

Guillermo E. Umpierrez

The primary goal of treatment of patients with type 1 diabetes mellitus (T1DM) or type 2 diabetes mellitus (T2DM) is to lower plasma glucose levels in order to prevent microvascular and macrovascular complications associated with chronic hyperglycemia. Improved glycemic control prevents the development and progression of diabetic complications. The Diabetes Control and Complications Trial (DCCT) reported that intensive insulin therapy in subjects with T1DM reduced the risk of developing retinopathy by 27% to 76%, nephropathy by 34% to 57%, and clinical neuropathy by 60% compared with conventional treatment.[1] In addition, intensive glycemic control reduced carotid intima-media thickness by 42% and risk of nonfatal myocardial infarction/stroke by 57%.[2] The U.K. Prospective Diabetes Study (UKPDS), a large randomized study in nearly 3900 patients with T2DM, showed that intensive treatment for over 10 years reduced by 25% the risk of microvascular complications compared with those who received conventional therapy.[3] In the UKPDS, each 1% reduction in Hb_{A1c} was associated with a 37% reduction in microvascular complications and a 21% reduction in any clinical event or death associated with diabetes. More recently, the European epidemiological diabetes study DECODE reported that elevated fasting plasma glucose and 2-hour postprandial glucose levels are associated with a significantly increased risk of cardiovascular mortality in T2DM.[4] Current guidelines from the American Diabetes Association recommend an Hb_{A1c} concentration less than 7%, a fasting plasma glucose level between 90 and 130 mg/dL (5.0 to 7.2 mmol/L), and a 2-hour postprandial plasma glucose less than 180 mg/dL (10 mmol/L).[5] Despite these guidelines, less than half of people with diabetes achieved recommended glycemic targets.[6]

Considerations for insulin initiation

Several factors need to be considered when selecting and managing candidates for insulin therapy, including type of diabetes, level of glycemic control, patient's motivation for optimizing glycemic control, and the availability of local resources to help patients adhere and adjust to the insulin regimen. Insulin therapy is the cornerstone of therapy in T1DM, as insulinopenia due to β-cell destruction requires insulin therapy for glycemic control and survival. Most patients with T2DM are managed with oral antidiabetic agents; however, patients can require insulin therapy during intercurrent illness (e.g., infection, acute medical illness), during a perioperative period, and with increased duration of diabetes and the resulting insulin deficiency from progressive β-cell failure. The type of insulin and route of administration, as well as the appropriate insulin dosage, is dependent on the glycemic response of the individual and glycemic control goals. Some poorly motivated patients or those with busy lifestyles may skip meals or be unwilling or unable to adhere to treatment regimens with complicated dosing or titration schedules. For these patients, simplified regimens may be beneficial, at least in the beginning of therapy. Glycemic targets need to be individualized for every patient and should take into account a patient's risk of developing microvascular complications. The pharmacokinetic variables of various insulins are summarized in Table 4.1.

Types of insulin

Short-acting insulin

Regular human insulin has an onset of action in 30 minutes, peaks at 2 to 3 hours when given subcutaneously, and has duration of action of 6 to 8 hours. It is a prandial insulin, but because of its delayed onset of action patients are instructed to inject regular insulin 20 to 30 minutes prior to meals.[7,8] Regular insulin has traditionally been used to target postprandial hyperglycemia and is used in combination with neutral protamine Hagedorn (NPH) and basal insulin.

Rapid-acting insulins

Rapid-acting insulin analogues differ from the regular human insulin in that certain amino acids in the insulin molecule are rearranged or substituted to modify the onset and duration of action.[9] There are three rapid-acting

Table 4.1 Available insulins in the United States				
Action	**Insulin type**	**Onset of action**	**Peak action**	**Duration of action**
Rapid-acting	Lispro, Aspart	5 to 15 min	45 min	3 to 4 h glulisine
Short-acting	Regular	15 to 30 min	2 to 3 h	4 to 6 h
Intermediate-acting	NPH	2 to 4 h	6 to 10 h	16 to 20 h
Long-acting	Glargine	3 to 4 h	No peak	20 to 24 h
	Detemir	3 to 4 h	No peak	14 to 20 h
Mixture				
NPH/regular	70/30, 50/50	30 min	Biphasic	16 to 20 h
NPH/lispro	75/25	5 to 15 min	Biphasic	16 to 20 h

Table 4.2 Recommendations for starting insulin therapy

Type 1 diabetes

- NPH and regular insulin regimen
  - Starting total daily dose (TDD): 0.3 to 0.5 IU/kg/day
  - Split-mixed insulin method (NPH and regular insulin): Give ⅔ of TDD before breakfast and ⅔ of TDD before dinner. Give ⅔ of the morning and evening dose as NPH and ⅓ as regular insulin.
  - Multidose insulin regimen: Give ⅔ of TDD before breakfast (⅔ NPH and ⅓ as regular insulin) and ⅓ of TDD in the evening, giving the regular insulin before dinner time and moving the NPH insulin from dinner to bedtime.
- Basal-bolus insulin regimen
  - Basal (glargine or detemir), rapid-acting insulin (lispro, aspart, glulisine) analogues
  - Starting TDD: 0.3 to 0.5 IU/kg/day
  - Give 50% of TDD as basal (glargine once/day; detemir once or twice daily) and 50% of TDD as rapid-acting analogue divided into 3 equal doses before meals

Type 2 diabetes

- Combination (add-on) insulin therapy to oral antidiabetic agents
  - NPH, glargine, or detemir at bedtime—starting TDD dose: 10 IU or 0.15 IU/kg in the evening
  - Increased TDD by 2 IU every 3 days to reach fasting blood glucose target (individualized for each patient, but usually <130 mg/dL)
- Split-mixed insulin method (starting TDD: 0.5 IU/kg/day): Give ⅔ of TDD before breakfast and ⅓ of TDD before dinner. Give ⅔ of the morning and evening dose as NPH and ⅓ as regular insulin.
- Basal-bolus insulin
  - Basal (glargine or detemir): 50% of TDD once daily, and bolus (lispro, aspart, glulisine) 50% of TDD before meals.
  - Increased basal insulin by 2 IU every 3 days to reach fasting and pre-meal blood glucose at target.

insulin analogues with similar pharmacokinetic profiles that are more suitable for targeting postprandial hyperglycemia: insulin lispro (Humalog), insulin aspart (Novolog), and insulin glulisine (Apidra). Lispro differs from regular insulin in that the 28th and 29th amino acids of the β chain of insulin are reversed to form lispro instead of pro-lys. Aspart is a recombinant human insulin in which aspartic acid is substituted for proline at B28. Glulisine has a lysine substituted for arginine at B3, and glutamic acid replaces lysine at B29. These insulin analogues are rapidly absorbed after subcutaneous injection (<30 minutes), peak at 1 hour, and have a duration of action of 3 to 4 hours.[8]

Several reports and meta-analyses have reported benefits with the use of rapid-acting insulin analogues in improving metabolic control and reducing the incidence of hypoglycemic episodes in patients with DM.[7] In a recent meta-analysis of 49 studies,10 adults with T1DM treated with rapid-acting insulin analogues had a small, but statistically significant, decrease in Hb_{A1c} compared with those treated with regular insulin. In patients with T2DM, however, no superiority in Hb_{A1c} reduction was observed. In terms of overall hypoglycemia, the results obtained with rapid-acting insulin analogues and with regular insulin were comparable.[10] One study[11] reported significantly less nocturnal hypoglycemic events requiring glucose or glucagon injection in patients with T1DM. The results in T2DM patients have been controversial, with some studies showing lower rates of nocturnal hypoglycemia and others reporting no statistically significant difference between the treatment arms.[10]

Intermediate-acting insulin

Intermediate-acting insulins, such as NPH insulin, have a delayed onset of action ranging between 2 and 4 hours and can take approximately 6 to 8 hours to reach peak concentration, and the duration of action can be up to 20 hours.[8] This leads to a distinct peak-and-trough effect, and therefore, when used as basal insulin, two or more injections are often required each day to minimize the daily excursions of insulin levels. Recently, production of lente insulin was discontinued because of decreasing market shares.

Basal insulins

Basal insulin preparations include glargine (Lantus) and detemir (Levemir) insulins (Fig. 4.1). Glargine has the addition of two arginines at the carboxy-terminal end of the β chain (B31 and B32) and the substitution of glycine for asparaginase at A21, which delays its solubility at physiological pH. Glargine has an onset of action of approximately 2 hours, reaches a plateau of biological action at 4 to 6 hours, and lasts up to 24 hours.[12] When insulin glargine became available, the recommended dosing interval was once daily at bedtime; however, it is approved for use at any time of day as long as it is administered at the same time each day. Insulin glargine has an acid pH (pH 4) and should not be mixed with any other insulin. Detemir is a basal insulin analogue that is soluble at neutral pH. After subcutaneous injection, insulin detemir binds to albumin through its fatty acid chain.[12,13] The mean duration of action of insulin detemir ranged from 5.7 hours at the lowest dose to 23.2 hours at the highest dose (sampling period 24 hours). Insulin detemir is therefore administered once or twice daily. As with insulin

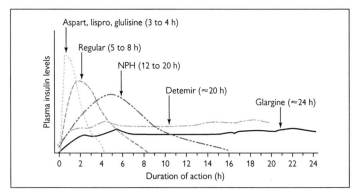

Figure 4.1 Time profiles of available insulin formulations.

glargine, insulin detemir has a more stable, less variable pharmacokinetic profile than does NPH. A recent meta-analysis of six studies comparing insulin glargine to NPH and two studies comparing insulin detemir to NPH insulin13 reported that metabolic control (measured by Hb_{A1c}) and adverse effects (hypoglycemia) did not differ between treatment groups. Although the overall rate of hypoglycemia rates was not different, the rate of symptomatic and nocturnal hypoglycemia were significantly lower in patients treated with glargine or detemir insulin.[13]

Premixed insulin formulations

There are two premixed conventional insulin formulations: Humulin 70/30 or Novolin 70/30, which consist of 70% NPH and 30% regular insulin, and Humulin 50/50, which consists of 50% NPH and 50% regular insulin. Conventional premixed human insulins have an onset of action of approximately 0.5 to 2 hours, usually plateau at 3 to 6 hours, and last up to 24 hours. Rapid-acting insulin analogues are also available in premixed preparations with rapid and intermediate insulin activity: Humalog mix 75/25, a 75% insulin lispro protamine suspension with 25% insulin lispro; Humalog mix 50/50, a 50% insulin lispro protamine suspension with 50% insulin lispro; and Novolog mix 70/30, a 70% insulin aspart protamine suspension with 30% insulin aspart. Insulin analogue mixes have an onset of action of approximately 15 minutes, reach a peak biological action at 1 to 4 hours, and last up to 24 hours. These insulins provide both prandial and basal activity for glycemic control. They are usually administered twice daily. Premixed fixed insulin preparations reduce the frequency of injections and have the convenience of the patient's not having to mix the respective insulin components prior to injection; however, they lack the flexibility of adjusting the respective insulin components with better precision for control of prandial glycemia and between meals/basal glycemia.

Insulin therapy in T1DM

The clinical presentation of patients with T1DM varies from mild to moderate polydipsia, polyuria, and fatigue to weight loss, dehydration, severe hyperglycemia, and diabetic ketoacidosis (DKA). In western European countries and the United States, about one-third to one-half of newly diagnosed children and adolescents present with the mild symptoms, and about one-third present with hyperglycemic crises. DKA is identified in approximately 40% of children and teenagers and in 17% of adults at the time of diagnosis of T1DM.[14] Patients with DKA are treated with intravenous regular insulin or with subcutaneous rapid-acting insulin analogues every 1 or 2 hours.[15–17] After hyperglycemia and ketosis are resolved, patients are treated with a multiple-dose insulin schedule combining regular or rapid-acting analogues and intermediate- or long-acting insulin. The starting total daily dose of insulin in patients with newly diagnosed diabetes is 0.6 IU/kg per day with daily titration until an optimal dose is established. Until recently, patients were treated with split-mixed insulin or a multidose insulin regimen of regular and intermediate-acting insulin (NPH). Recently, regimens using long-acting basal and rapid-acting prandial insulin have been suggested as a more physiological approach to glucose control in the hospital[18,19] and to facilitate outpatient glycemic control with lower rate of hypoglycemic events than NPH/regular insulin.[20–23]

Newly diagnosed T1DM without ketoacidosis is best treated with a combination of basal and rapid-acting insulin taken before meals. The total daily dose of insulin in patients with T1DM should be started at 0.3 to 0.5 IU/kg. In most patients with established disease, the total daily insulin dose ranges between 0.6 and 0.9 units/kg body weight.[1] The newer insulin analogues given as basal (glargine or detemir) once daily and bolus (lispro, aspart, or glulisine) before each meal have been shown to be associated with improved glycemic control with a lower rate of hypoglycemia.[24,25] Achieving glycemic targets in T1DM with conventional twice-daily (NPH and regular) insulins is difficult and is associated with increased risk of hypoglycemia.[1,24] Multidose insulin (MDI) therapy using multiple injections (more than three) per day is frequently needed for optimal diabetes control in patients with T1DM. Moving the NPH insulin from dinner time to bedtime and continuing with mixed NPH and regular insulin in the morning and regular insulin before dinner time has been shown to be effective in improving glycemic control with a low rate of hypoglycemic events compared to traditional split-mixed insulin regimen with NPH and regular insulin twice daily.[26,27]

Continuous subcutaneous insulin infusion (CSII) with an infusion pump is another valid alternative to conventional injection therapy for achieving glycemic control. Patients with T1DM receiving CSII therapy show more improvement in Hb_{A1c} levels and a lower rate of hypoglycemic events than do patients receiving intensive multiple insulin injections.[28] CSII provides increased flexibility in dosing and may improve quality of life in some patients. A meta-analysis of the studies evaluating the efficacy and safety of insulin pump therapy has found a modest advantage of this approach compared with multiple-dose insulin injection protocols.[29] Patients treated with CSII use less insulin; it is recommended to decrease the total daily dose of subcutaneous insulin by 20% to 30% and then use 50% of that reduced dose as basal insulin.[24] Rapid-acting analogues are the preferred insulin formulation and improved prandial control compared to regular insulin.

Insulin therapy in type 2 diabetes mellitus

The most common indication for long-term insulin therapy in T2DM is in patients who have experienced primary or secondary failure to oral antidiabetic therapy. For patients with inadequate glycemic control with oral antidiabetic agents, the addition of NPH insulin at bedtime or insulin glargine or detemir at anytime during the day effectively lowers glycemia. In the Treat-to-Target study,[21] subjects who were not at target Hb_{A1c} while taking one to two oral antidiabetic agents received add-on therapy with NPH or glargine at bedtime. More than 55% of subjects treated with either NPH or glargine insulin achieved the target Hb_{A1c} of <7%; however, those treated with glargine had lower frequency of nocturnal hypoglycemia. A similar reduction in hypoglycemic events has been reported with insulin detemir compared to NPH as add-on therapy to oral agents in T2DM.[30] About one-third of patients treated with detemir insulin require the dose of detemir to be given twice daily in order to improve glycemic control.

The starting basal insulin dose as add-on therapy to T2DM patients who have failed to achieve glycemic control with oral antidiabetic agents is 10 IU/day or 0.15 IU/kg per day. The average daily insulin dose in clinical trials is about 40 to 50 IU/day.[21] Thus, the daily insulin dose should be adjusted periodically to achieve glycemic control. Patients with diabetes should be instructed not only in insulin administration but also in self-adjustment of their daily insulin dose. When adjustment algorithms are simplified, many patients are able to effectively and safely self-titrate their bedtime basal insulin dose. This was demonstrated in the ATLANTUS study in which patients were given instructions to self-adjust their basal insulin dose by 2 units every 3 days to achieve blood glucose levels <120 mg/dL.[31] In this study, patients achieved target Hb_{A1c} levels more often using a patient-driven algorithm versus a weekly physician-driven titration. Patients managed with basal insulin therapy alone with high fasting glucose and Hb_{A1c} levels should be started on basal and prandial insulin combination.

Complications of insulin therapy

Hypoglycemia is the most dreaded complication of using insulin, particularly for those on intensive regimens. The recent American Diabetes Association workgroup on hypoglycemia defined *hypoglycemia* as an event during which typical symptoms of hypoglycemia are accompanied by a measured plasma glucose concentration <70 mg/dL (3.9 mmol/L).[32] *Severe hypoglycemia* is defined as an event requiring the assistance of another person to actively administer carbohydrate, glucagon, or other resuscitative actions. Hypoglycemia occurs approximately once or twice weekly in patients with T1DM receiving intensive treatment. The prevalence of hypoglycemia in patients with T2DM varies according to the type of therapy. A higher prevalence of hypoglycemia is reported in patients treated with insulin than in those treated with oral agents. The risk of hypoglycemia is lower with long-acting insulin glargine[21] and insulin detemir[30] compared with NPH and premixed insulins. Rapid-acting insulin analogues are also associated with a lower frequency of hypoglycemia compared with regular insulins.[33]

Recurrent episodes of hypoglycemia may result in the loss of recognition of early-warning or autonomic symptoms, and patients may remain asymptomatic even when plasma glucose is very low. This condition, labeled hypoglycemia-associated autonomic failure, is common in T1DM but also occurs in T2DM.[34] In the DCCT, 60% of severe hypoglycemic episodes occurred without warning, especially at night. Such patients are not candidates for tight glycemic control, but, fortunately, the hypoglycemia unawareness can be alleviated after a period of several weeks to months through careful avoidance of further episodes. General guidelines for the management of hypoglycemia in patients with diabetes is shown in Table 4.3.

Table 4.3 Management of hypoglycemia in patients with diabetes

1. Recognize cause of hypoglycemia risk
   - Hypoglycemia unawareness
   - Missed meals or reduced food intake
   - Strenuous or unplanned exercise
   - Excess alcohol intake
   - Stress
   - Comorbid disease (renal failure, panhypopituitarism, hypothyroidism)

2. Reducing the risk of hypoglycemia
   - Patient education
   - Encourage self-monitoring
   - Set appropriate goal setting (avoid tight control in patients with hypoglycemic unawareness, renal failure, adrenal insufficiency, panhypopituitarism)
   - Encourage limited alcohol consumption
   - Emphasize balanced food intake
   - Carry fast-acting carbohydrate

3. Treatment
   - Mild to moderate hypoglycemia (blood glucose <70 mg/dL, minimal or no symptoms)
     - Fast-acting carbohydrates (25 g) as glucose tablets, fruit juices, or high-sugar drinks
     - Repeat carbohydrate snack if plasma glucose remains <70 mg/dL 15 minutes later
   - Severe hypoglycemia (blood glucose <40 mg/dL, neuroglycopenia)
     - IV administration of glucose (25 g)
     - Glucagon 1 mg subcutaneous or intramuscular

Besides increasing the risk for hypoglycemia, there are a few additional side effects of insulin. Insulin use is associated with weight gain. In the DCCT trial, the patients on intensive insulin regimens gained 5.1 kg versus 2.4 kg in those on conventional therapy. In the UKPDS study, those on insulin gained 10.4 kg versus 3.7 kg for those using sulfonylureas. Local and systemic allergic reactions to insulin are rare with the use of human insulins and analogues as the purity of the product has improved. There seems to be a genetic predisposition to insulin allergy. Studies have shown that insulin antibodies are more likely to form if a patient is HLA-Bw44 and DR7 or B15 or DR4 than those with B8 and DR3. Lipodystrophy of subcutaneous tissues is an immunologic response to insulin that results from repeated insulin injection into one site. Serious insulin reactions, including anaphylaxis, generalized urticaria, or angioedema, are very rare and can be mediated through IgE antibodies. Desensitization techniques are then used to allow use of insulin. Worsening of diabetic retinopathy during the first year of improved glycemic control in persons with underlying retinopathy has been reported in approximately 5% of patients.[24,35] Patients with proliferative retinopathy with an Hb_{A1c} greater than 10% are at highest risk of worsening retinopathy. In such patients, it is recommended to reduce the Hb_{A1c} levels slowly (2% per year) with frequent ophthalmologic examinations and treatment as needed.[24] After 5 to 7 years of improved blood sugar levels, the degree of retinopathy is less severe than in those with continued uncontrolled glucoses.

In summary, patients with T1DM almost always require insulin to achieve the recommended Hb_{A1c} target level of <7%. In such patients, multidose insulin injections with insulin analogues have proved to be more effective than conventional human insulins. They also provide more flexibility and are associated with significant reduction in the rate of hypoglycemic events. In subjects with T2DM, the timely addition of insulin to oral therapy has been shown to be effective and safe (i.e., fewer hypoglycemic episodes), providing for a once-daily dosing and mimicking the physiological secretory profile of endogenous insulin. A variety of insulin preparations with different profiles are available, allowing for individualized regimens for optimal glycemic control.

References

1. The Diabetes Control and Complications Trial Research Group. The effect of intensive treatment of diabetes on the development and progression of long-term complications in insulin-dependent diabetes mellitus. *N Engl J Med.* 1993;329:977–986.

2. Nathan DM, Cleary PA, Backlund JY, et al. Intensive diabetes treatment and cardiovascular disease in patients with type 1 diabetes. *N Engl J Med.* 2005;353:2643–2653.

3. UK Prospective Diabetes Study (UKPDS) Group. Intensive blood-glucose control with sulphonylureas or insulin compared with conventional treatment and risk of complications in patients with type 2 diabetes (UKPDS 33). *Lancet.* 1998;352:837–853.

4. Is the current definition for diabetes relevant to mortality risk from all causes and cardiovascular and noncardiovascular diseases? *Diabetes Care.* 2003;26:688–696.

5. Standards of medical care in diabetes—2008. *Diabetes Care.* 2008;31(suppl 1): S12–S54.

6. Koro CE, Bowlin SJ, Bourgeois N, Fedder DO. Glycemic control from 1988 to 2000 among U.S. adults diagnosed with type 2 diabetes: a preliminary report. *Diabetes Care.* 2004;27:17–20.

7. Gulan M, Gottesman IS, Zinman B. Biosynthetic human insulin improves postprandial glucose excursions in type I diabetics. *Ann Intern Med.* 1987;107:506–509.

8. Mooradian AD, Bernbaum M, Albert SG. Narrative review: a rational approach to starting insulin therapy. *Ann Intern Med.* 2006;145:125–134.

9. Salsali A, Nathan M. A review of types 1 and 2 diabetes mellitus and their treatment with insulin. *Am J Ther.* 2006;13:349–361.

10. Siebenhofer A, Plank J, Berghold A, et al. Short-acting insulin analogues versus regular human insulin in patients with diabetes mellitus. *Cochrane Database Syst Rev.* 2006;CD003287.

11. Home PD, Lindholm A, Riis A. Insulin aspart vs. human insulin in the management of long-term blood glucose control in type 1 diabetes mellitus: a randomized controlled trial. *Diabet Med.* 2000;17:762–770.

12. Edelman SV, Morello CM. Strategies for insulin therapy in type 2 diabetes. *South Med J.* 2005;98:363–371.

13. Horvath K, Jeitler K, Berghold A, et al. Long-acting insulin analogues versus NPH insulin (human isophane insulin) for type 2 diabetes mellitus. *Cochrane Database Syst Rev.* 2007;CD005613.

14. Kaufman FR, Halvorson M. The treatment and prevention of diabetic keto-acidosis in children and adolescents with type I diabetes mellitus. *Pediatr Ann.* 1999;28:576–582.

15. Kitabchi AE, Umpierrez GE, Murphy MB, Kreisberg RA. Hyperglycemic crises in adult patients with diabetes: a consensus statement from the American Diabetes Association. *Diabetes Care.* 2006;29:2739–2748.

16. Umpierrez GE, Cuervo R, Karabell A, Latif K, Freire AX, Kitabchi AE. Treatment of diabetic ketoacidosis with subcutaneous insulin aspart. *Diabetes Care.* 2004;27:1873–1878.

17. Umpierrez GE, Latif K, Stoever J, et al. Efficacy of subcutaneous insulin lispro versus continuous intravenous regular insulin for the treatment of patients with diabetic ketoacidosis. *Am J Med.* 2004;117:291–296.

18. Clement S, Braithwaite SS, Magee MF, et al. Management of diabetes and hyper-glycemia in hospitals. *Diabetes Care.* 2004;27:553–597.

19. Inzucchi SE. Clinical practice. Management of hyperglycemia in the hospital setting. *N Engl J Med.* 2006;355:1903–1911.

20. Gerich JE. Insulin glargine: long-acting basal insulin analog for improved meta-bolic control. *Curr Med Res Opin.* 2004;20:31–37.

21. Riddle MC, Rosenstock J, Gerich J. The treat-to-target trial: randomized addition of glargine or human NPH insulin to oral therapy of type 2 diabetic patients. *Diabetes Care.* 2003;26:3080–3086.

22. Kiess W, Raile K, Galler A, Kapellen T. Insulin detemir offers improved glycemic control compared with NPH insulin in people with type 1 diabetes. *Diabetes Care.* 2004;27:2567–2568.

23. Hermansen K, Madsbad S, Perrild H, Kristensen A, Axelsen M. Comparison of the soluble basal insulin analog insulin detemir with NPH insulin: a randomized open crossover trial in type 1 diabetic subjects on basal-bolus therapy. *Diabetes Care.* 2001;24:296–301.

24. DeWitt DE, Hirsch IB. Outpatient insulin therapy in type 1 and type 2 diabetes mellitus: scientific review. *JAMA.* 2003;289:2254–2264.

25. Gale EA. A randomized, controlled trial comparing insulin lispro with human soluble insulin in patients with type 1 diabetes on intensified insulin therapy. The UK Trial Group. *Diabet Med.* 2000;17:209–214.

26. Francis AJ, Home PD, Hanning I, Alberti KG, Tunbridge WM. Intermediate act-ing insulin given at bedtime: effect on blood glucose concentrations before and after breakfast. *Br Med J (Clin Res Ed).* 1983;286:1173–1176.

27. Fanelli CG, Pampanelli S, Porcellati F, Rossetti P, Brunetti P, Bolli GB. Administration of neutral protamine Hagedorn insulin at bedtime versus with dinner in type 1 diabetes mellitus to avoid nocturnal hypoglycemia and improve control. A randomized, controlled trial. *Ann Intern Med.* 2002;136:504–514.

28. Pickup J, Mattock M, Kerry S. Glycaemic control with continuous subcutaneous insulin infusion compared with intensive insulin injections in patients with type 1 diabetes: meta-analysis of randomised controlled trials. *BMJ.* 2002;324:705.

29. Retnakaran R, Hochman J, DeVries JH, et al. Continuous subcutaneous insulin infusion versus multiple daily injections: the impact of baseline A1c. *Diabetes Care.* 2004;27:2590–2596.

30. Hermansen K, Davies M, Derezinski T, Martinez Ravn G, Clauson P, Home P. A 26-week, randomized, parallel, treat-to-target trial comparing insulin detemir with NPH insulin as add-on therapy to oral glucose-lowering drugs in insulin-naive people with type 2 diabetes. *Diabetes Care*. 2006;29:1269–1274.

31. Davies M, Storms F, Shutler S, Bianchi-Biscay M, Gomis R. Improvement of glycemic control in subjects with poorly controlled type 2 diabetes: comparison of two treatment algorithms using insulin glargine. *Diabetes Care*. 2005;28:1282–1288.

32. Defining and reporting hypoglycemia in diabetes: a report from the American Diabetes Association Workgroup on Hypoglycemia. *Diabetes Care*. 2005;28:1245–1249.

33. Bastyr EJ 3rd, Huang Y, Brunelle RL, Vignati L, Cox DJ, Kotsanos JG. Factors associated with nocturnal hypoglycaemia among patients with type 2 diabetes new to insulin therapy: experience with insulin lispro. *Diabetes Obes Metab*. 2000;2:39–46.

34. Cryer PE, Davis SN, Shamoon H. Hypoglycemia in diabetes. *Diabetes Care*. 2003;26:1902–1912.

35. Helve E, Laatikainen L, Merenmies L, Koivisto VA. Continuous insulin infusion therapy and retinopathy in patients with type I diabetes. *Acta Endocrinol (Copenh)*. 1987;115:313–319.

Chapter 5

Diabetes complications

Vivian Fonseca

The hallmark of diabetes is its long-term complications, which are a significant cause of morbidity and mortality worldwide. In this chapter, we discuss strategies to detect complications early and to treat them or their symptoms early in order to slow their progression and/or improve the quality of life of patients. Most of these recommendations are consistent with the standards of care of the American Diabetes Association and other organizations, and most are based on evidence from clinical trials.[1]

Microvascular complications

Microvascular complications (listed in Table 5.1) are specific for diabetes and are almost certainly related to hyperglycemia. Hyperglycemia leads to multiple biochemical changes that cause tissue damage, some of which are listed in Table 5.1.[2] These lead to changes in various organs, as summarized in Figure 5.1. Most of these changes can be prevented by good glycemic control, which prevents the development of the complications and slows their progression.[3] There is a very good correlation between Hb_{A1c} and microvascular complication, but the relationship is less linear with macrovascular events (Fig. 5.1).[4] Indeed, clinical trials have demonstrated a reduction in the risk of microvascular, but not macrovascular, complications with improved glycemic control. However, attempts to achieve a normal Hb_{A1c} in the ACCORD trial[5] led to an increased risk of all-cause mortality and should therefore be attempted with caution in high-risk patients. However, other important clinical trials are ongoing, and the results may help clarify this important issue.

Diabetic retinopathy

Diabetic retinopathy is estimated to be the most frequent cause of new cases of blindness among adults aged 20 to 74 years. Glaucoma, cataracts, and other disorders of the eye also occur earlier and more frequently in people with diabetes. Screening recommendations in adults with type 1 diabetes mellitus (T1DM) include an initial dilated and comprehensive eye examination within 5 years of the diagnosis of diabetes. Adults with type 2

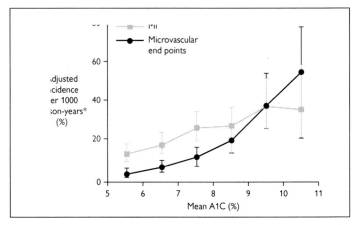

Figure 5.1 Relationship between HbA1c and microvascular and macrovascular complications. Reprinted from Stratton IM et al., *BMJ*. 2000:321:405–412, with permission from BMJ Publishing Group, Ltd. © 2000. All rights reserved.
MI = myocardial infarction.
* Adjusted for age, sex, and ethnic group; white men aged 50 to 54 y at diagnosis; mean duration of diagnosis of 10 y.

Table 5.1 Molecular and physiological effects of hyperglycemia that contribute to long-term complications
• Glycation of proteins (e.g., hemoglobin, collagen, LDL, cholesterol)
• Accumulation of sorbitol and fructose (e.g., in nerves, lens)
• Activation of protein kinase C and aldose reductase
• Formation of altered proteins (glycation end products)
• Cytokine activation
• Oxidative stress
• Increased osmotic load in tissues
• Acute reduction motor and sensory nerve conduction velocity
• Increased glomerular filtration rate and renal plasma flow

Table 5.2 Impact of tight metabolic control on complications

Hb$_{A1c}$	DCCT 9% to 7%	Kumamoto 9% to 7%	UKPDS 8% to 7%	ACCORD 7.5% to 6.4%	ADVANCE 7.5% to 6.5%
Retinopathy	↓ 63%	↓ 69%	↓ 17% to 21%		
Nephropathy	↓ 54%–70%	↓	↓ 24% to 33%		↓ Decreased
Neuropathy	↓ 60%	Improved			
Macrovascular disease	↓ 41%		↓ 16%*#	↓ 10%*	↓ 10%*
Mortality			↓@	↑	

* Not statistically significant;
# Significant on long-term follow up.
@ Significant with metformin only but significant with SU and Insulin on follow up.
Reprinted with permission from Fonseca, Pendergrass, and McDuffie. *Handbook of Diabetes*. Current Medicine Group © 2008.

Table 5.3 Summary of the risk reduction profiles of various treatments for blood pressure, lipids, and glucose on microvascular and macrovascular events

Treatment	Microvascular events	Macrovascular events
Blood pressure treatment	20% to 40%	20% to 50%
Lipid treatment	—	25% to 55%
Glucose treatment	12% to 35%*	10% to 20%*

*Per 1% A1C reduction.

Reprinted with permission from Fonseca, Pendergrass, and McDuffie. *Handbook of Diabetes.* Current Medicine Group © 2008.

Table 5.4 Goals for diabetic retinopathy

- Optimal glucose and blood pressure control
- Dilated and comprehensive eye examination by an ophthalmologist or optometrist within 3 to 5 years after the onset of type 1 diabetes and shortly after diagnosis of type 2; subsequent examinations should be repeated annually by an ophthalmologist or optometrist
- Fundus photography may be a useful alternative screening tool
- Pregnancy is associated with worsening of retinopathy; eye examination should occur in the first trimester with close follow-up throughout pregnancy and for 1 year postpartum
- Laser therapy can reduce the risk of vision loss in patients with high-risk characteristics
- Intraorbital steroids can help reduce macular edema

diabetes mellitus (T2DM) should have an initial dilated and comprehensive eye examination shortly following the diagnosis of diabetes. Subsequent examinations for patients with T1DM or T2DM should be repeated annually. Examinations will be required more frequently if retinopathy is progressing or in anyone with a change or loss of vision.

Intensive diabetes management with the goal of achieving near normoglycemia prevents/delays the onset of diabetic retinopathy.[3,6,7] In addition to glycemic control, several other factors seem to increase the risk of retinopathy. High blood pressure is a risk factor for the development of macular edema and is associated with the presence of proliferative diabetic retinopathy (PDR). Studies have shown a reduction in the risk of retinopathy with good blood pressure control. In T1DM patients, retinopathy has been reported to deteriorate.

Examinations also can be done using retinal photographs (with or without dilation of the pupil) and having these read by experienced experts in this field. In older-onset patients with severe nonproliferative diabetic retinopathy or less-than-high-risk PDR, the risk of severe visual loss and vitrectomy is reduced by laser photocoagulation. Laser photocoagulation surgery is beneficial in reducing the risk of further visual loss but generally is not beneficial in reversing already diminished acuity.

Diabetic nephropathy

Diabetic nephropathy occurs in almost 40% of patients with diabetes and is the single leading cause of end-stage renal disease (ESRD). Albuminuria in the range of 30 to 299 mg/24 h is called microalbuminuria. Persistent microalbuminuria is the earliest clinical evidence of nephropathy as well as a marker of cardiovascular complications in diabetes. Analysis of a spot sample for the albumin-to-creatinine ratio is the best screening test. Microalbuminuria is a well-established marker of increased cerebrovascular disease (CVD) risk.[8,9] Patients with microalbuminuria who progress to macroalbuminuria (>300 mg/24 h) are likely to progress to ESRD. Several interventions have been demonstrated to reduce the risk and slow the progression of renal disease. Blockade of the renin-angiotensin-aldosterone system (RAAS) with angiotensin-converting enzyme inhibitors (ACEIs) and angiotensin II receptor blockers (ARBs) is the most effective approach in treating nephropathy.

Intensive diabetes and blood pressure management have been shown in large prospective randomized studies to delay the onset of microalbuminuria and the progression of microalbuminuria to macroalbuminuria in patients with T1DM or T2DM. In addition, ACEIs and ARBs have been shown to reduce severe CVD (i.e., myocardial infarction, stroke, death). Although combining these classes of drugs leads to further reduction in proteinuria, the combination has no impact on outcomes.

Serum creatinine should be measured at least annually for the estimation of glomerular filtration rate (GFR) in all adults with diabetes, regardless of the degree of urine albumin excretion. Serum creatinine alone should not be used as a measure of kidney function but should be used to estimate GFR and stage the level of chronic kidney disease. The Cockcroft-Gault equation is commonly used to estimate GFR:

$$[(140 - Age [years]) \times Body Weight (kg) \times k]/Serum Creatinine (\mu mol/L)$$

where k is a constant: 1.23 (males) or 1.04 (females). Normal range is >90 mL/min, and mild, moderate, and severe renal dysfunction are defined as

Table 5.5 Diagnosing and treating diabetic nephropathy	
• Screen for microalbuminuria	
Category	**Spot collection (μg/mg creatinine)**
Normal	<30
Microalbuminuria	30 to 299
Macro (clinical)-albuminuria	≥300
• In the treatment of both microalbuminuria and macroalbuminuria, either ACE inhibitors or ARBs should be used, except during pregnancy.	
• Monitor serum potassium levels for the development of hyperkalemia. Good blood pressure control is critical in nephropathy management. Multiple drugs may be needed.	

Table 5.6 Stages of chronic kidney disease		
Stage	**Description**	**GFR (mL/min per 1.73 m²body surface area)**
1	Kidney damage with normal or increased GFR	>90
2	Kidney damage with mildly decreased GFR	60 to 89
3	Moderately decreased GFR	30 to 59
4	Severely decreased GFR	15 to 29
5	Kidney failure	<15 or dialysis

GFR, glomerular filtration rate.
Reprinted with permission from Fonseca, Pendergrass, and McDuffie. *Handbook of Diabetes.* Current Medicine Group © 2008.

a GFR of 60 to 90 mL/min, 30 to 60 mL/min, and 15 to 30 mL/min, respectively. Patients with end-stage renal disease have a GFR of <15 mL/min. Referral to a renal specialist should be considered when the estimated GFR has fallen to <60 mL/min or if difficulties occur in the management of hypertension or hyperkalemia. The estimated GFR can easily be calculated using the program at the National Kidney Foundation's Web site (http://www.kidney.org/professionals/kdoqi/gfr_calculator.cfm).

Diabetic neuropathy

The term *diabetic neuropathy* encompasses a wide range of conditions with diverse clinical manifestations.[10] The most common clinical presentation is chronic sensorimotor distal symmetric polyneuropathy (DPN) and autonomic neuropathy. Although DPN is a diagnosis of exclusion, complex investigations to exclude other conditions are rarely needed.[10]

Patients with diabetes should be screened annually for DPN using tests such as pinprick sensation; temperature; vibration perception (using a 128 Hz tuning fork); 10 g monofilament pressure sensation at the dorsal surface of both great toes, just proximal to the nail bed; and ankle reflexes. Combinations of more than one test have >87% sensitivity in detecting DPN. Loss of 10 g monofilament perception and reduced vibration perception predict foot ulcers. A minimum of one clinical test should be carried out annually.

Foot care

Amputation and foot ulceration are the most common consequences of diabetic neuropathy and major causes of morbidity and disability in people with diabetes. Early recognition and management of independent risk factors can prevent or delay adverse outcomes.

Table 5.7 Symptoms of peripheral neuropathy

Positive symptoms	Negative symptoms
Burning pain	Feet are asleep/"dead"
Knife-like	Numbness
Electrical sensations	Tingling/prickling
Squeezing	
Constricting	
Freezing	
Throbbing	
Allodynia	

Table 5.8 Goals for neuropathy

- Screen at diagnosis and at least annually thereafter. Use vibration/temperature sense and reflexes.
- If positive:
  - Assess for risk of ulcer/amputation:monofilament test, deformity, toe nail dystrophy, callus, dry skin.
- Special foot care is appropriate for insensate feet to decrease the risk of amputation.
- Simple inspection of insensate feet should be performed at 3- to 6-month intervals. An abnormality should trigger referral for special footwear, preventive specialist, or podiatric care.
- Education of patients about self-care of the feet and referral for special shoes/ inserts.

Table 5.9 Conditions associated with an increased risk of amputation

- Peripheral neuropathy with loss of sensation
- Diabetes >10 years, poor glucose control, presence of other diabetes complications
- Evidence of increased pressure (erythema, hemorrhage under a callus)
- Bony deformity
- Peripheral vascular disease (decreased or absent pedal pulses)
- History of ulcers or amputation
- Severe nail pathology
- Charcot joints

Reprinted with permission from Fonseca, Pendergrass, and McDuffie. *Handbook of Diabetes.* Current Medicine Group © 2008.

Symptomatic treatments

There is no approved treatment that alters the natural course of diabetic neuropathy. However, it is important to provide patients with symptomatic relief, particularly when pain is a major symptom.[10,11] Approaches to this problem are summarized in Table 5.12.

Table 5.10 Preventive foot care

- Comprehensive foot examination and foot self-care education.
- Use of a monofilament, tuning fork, palpation, and visual examination.
- A multidisciplinary approach is recommended for individuals with foot ulcers and high-risk feet, especially those with a history of prior ulcer or amputation.
- Refer patients with prior lower extremity complications to foot care specialists for ongoing preventive care and lifelong surveillance.
- Screening for peripheral arterial disease (PAD) history of claudication and an assessment of the pedal pulses. Consider obtaining an ankle-brachial index (ABI).

Table 5.11 Management of foot ulcers

- Involve specialist in foot care—podiatry, orthopedics, etc.
- Local healing factors (e.g., platelet-derived growth factor, etc.) along with debridement and keeping ulcer free of infection
- Total contact cast
- Achilles tendon lengthening
- Look for osteomyelitis—MRI, bone scan
- Amputation when appropriate, followed by quick rehabilitation

Stable and optimal glycemic control may help some patients and will slow the progression of disease. However, some patients get worsening of pain with sudden improvement in control. Commonly used treatments for pain include *tricyclic drugs*—amitriptyline and imipramine—although they do not have formal U.S. Food and Drug Administration (FDA) approval for this condition. The side effects limit their use in many patients. Tricyclic drugs may also exacerbate some autonomic symptoms such as gastroparesis. In addition, anticonvulsants like gabapentin have been used to treat pain. Pregabalin is longer acting, has also been confirmed to be useful in painful diabetic neuropathy, and is approved for use in this condition. Other anticonvulsant drugs may also be efficacious in the management of neuropathic pain. The 5-hydroxytryptamine (serotonin)-norepinephrine reuptake inhibitor duloxetine has been approved by the FDA for the treatment of neuropathic pain.

Diabetic autonomic neuropathy

The symptoms of autonomic dysfunction should be elicited carefully during the history and review of systems, particularly because many of these symptoms are potentially treatable.[10] Major clinical manifestations of diabetic autonomic neuropathy include resting tachycardia, exercise

Table 5.12 Treatment of painful diabetic neuropathy

Approach	Treatment type/drug	Dose per day	Remarks
Optimal diabetes control	Diet, OAD, insulin	Individual adaptation	Aim: $Hb_{A1c} \leq 7\%$
Symptomatic treatment	**Tricyclic antidepressants**		
	Amitriptyline	25 to 150 mg	Other tricyclics also work
	SSNRI		
	Duloxetine	60 to 120 mg	Nausea, rise in Hb_{A1c} (small)
	Anticonvulsants		
	Gabapentin	900 to 3600 mg	High doses needed
	Pregabalin	300 to 600 mg	Weight gain
	Carbamazepine	200 to 600 mg	Poor data quality
	Weak opioids		
	Tramadol	50 to 400 mg	Addictive
	Local treatment		
	Capsaicin (0.025%) cream	qid topically	Maximum duration: 6 to 8 wk
	Strong opioids		
Pain resistant to standard pharmacotherapy	Oxycodone		Highly addictive
	Electrical spinal cord stimulation		Invasive, specialist required
Physical therapy	TENS, EMS, medical gymnastics		No AEs
	Acupuncture		Uncontrolled study
	Psychological support		
Alternative treatments	α-Lipoić acid, Evening Primrose Oil	Variable	Proven to work in clinical trials
	Clonidine	Oral or skin patch	

intolerance, orthostatic hypotension, constipation, gastroparesis, erectile dysfunction, sudomotor dysfunction, impaired neurovascular function, "brittle diabetes," and hypoglycemic autonomic failure.

Gastrointestinal disturbances (e.g., gastroparesis, constipation/diarrhea, fecal incontinence) are common, and any section of the gastrointestinal tract may be affected. Gastroparesis should be suspected in individuals with erratic glucose control. Investigative test results often correlate poorly with symptoms.

Common features of autonomic neuropathy and their treatment are summarized in Table 5.13.

Table 5.13 Features of autonomic neuropathy and their treatment

System affected	Features	Treatment
Cardiovascular	Arrhythmias, sudden death	
	Orthostatic hypotension	Sodium chloride, fludrocortisone, ProAmatine
Gastrointestinal	Gastroparesis	Metoclopramide, cisapride, erythromycin
	Diarrhea	Loperamide, tetracyclines, clonidine, octreotide
Genitourinary	Erectile dysfunction	PDE5 inhibitors, vacuum pump, prostaglandins, prosthesis
	Incontinence—urinary	Bethanechol chloride, oxybutynin, self-catheterization

Macrovascular complications

CVD is the major cause of mortality for individuals with diabetes. It is also a major contributor to morbidity and direct and indirect costs of diabetes. T2DM is an independent risk factor for macrovascular disease, and its common coexisting conditions (e.g., hypertension and dyslipidemia) are also risk factors.

Extensive evidence from clinical trials suggests that broad-based treatment of hypertension, dyslipidemia, and hypercoagulability can improve clinical outcome and prevent cerebrovascular events in people with diabetes. In the Steno-2 study, a multiple-risk-factor reduction approach led to reduction in CVD events and, on follow-up, to a reduction in mortality.[12,13] Figure 5.2 illustrates the results from that trial. In addition, obesity, insulin resistance, and other risk factors may play a role.

Obesity—in particular, visceral or intraabdominal obesity—leads to insulin resistance and an increase in free fatty acids and inflammatory cytokines. This progresses to the development of not only diabetes but also other associated factors, including dyslipidemia (low HDL cholesterol, elevated triglycerides, and an increase in small-density LDL particles), hypertension, impaired clot breakdown (manifested as an elevation in plasminogen activator inhibitor-1 [PAI-1]), enhanced platelet aggregation, endothelial dysfunction, inflammation, and microalbuminuria.[14] Table 5.14 summarizes some of these "nontraditional" risk factors for CVD.

Hypertension/blood pressure control

Hypertension (blood pressure >140/90 mmHg) is a common comorbidity of diabetes, affecting the majority of people with diabetes (particularly T2DM), depending on type of diabetes, age, obesity, and ethnicity. Hypertension is

Table 5.14 Nontraditional risk factors for cerebrovascular disease in patients with diabetes

Established risk factors
- Hypertension
- Lipids
- Obesity
- Smoking

Nontraditional risk factors
- Insulin resistance
- Abnormal fibrinolysis—PAI-1
- Endothelial dysfunction
- Microalbuminuria
- Markers of inflammation—CRP
- Vascular wall abnormalities
- Homocysteine
- Hypercoagulation
- Postprandial hyperglycemia

CRP, C-reactive protein.

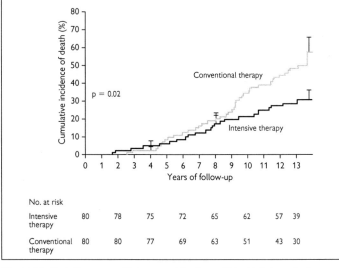

Figure 5.2 Mortality compared between an intensive multiple risk factor reduction approach with a control group (13). Gaede P, Lund-Andersen H, Parving HH, Pedersen O. Effect of a multifactorial intervention on mortality in type 2 diabetes. *N Engl J Med*. 2008 Feb 7;358(6):580–91. Copyright © 2008, Massachusetts Medical Society. All rights reserved.

Table 5.15 Managing blood pressure to goal in diabetes

- Blood pressure should be measured at every routine diabetes visit.
- Goals: systolic blood pressure <130 mmHg and diastolic blood pressure <80 mmHg.
- Multiple drug therapy (two or more agents at proper doses) is generally required to achieve blood pressure targets.
- Blockade of the renin-angiotensin system improves outcomes over and above what can be expected from blood pressure reduction alone.
- ACE inhibitors and angiotensin receptor blockers (ARBs) have been shown to delay the progression of nephropathy.

also a major risk factor for CVD and microvascular complications such as retinopathy and nephropathy.

Lowering of blood pressure with regimens based on antihypertensive drugs, including ACEIs, ARBs, β-blockers, diuretics, and calcium channel blockers, has been shown to be effective in lowering cardiovascular events.

ACEIs have been shown to improve cardiovascular outcomes in high-cardiovascular-risk patients with or without hypertension. In patients with congestive heart failure (CHF), the addition of ARBs to either ACEIs or other therapies reduces the risk of cardiovascular death or hospitalization for heart failure. However, the Antihypertensive and Lipid-Lowering Treatment to Prevent Heart Attack Trial (ALLHAT), a large randomized trial of different initial blood pressure pharmacological therapies, found no large differences between initial therapy with a chlorthalidone, amlodipine, and lisinopril. There were no differences between ACEIs and ARBs.

Lipids

Patients with T2DM have an increased prevalence of lipid abnormalities that contributes to higher rates of CVD. Lipid management aimed at lowering LDL cholesterol, raising HDL cholesterol, and lowering triglycerides has been shown to reduce macrovascular disease and mortality in patients with T2DM, particularly in those who have had prior cardiovascular events. In studies using HMG (hydroxymethylglutaryl)-CoA reductase inhibitors (statins), patients with diabetes achieved significant reductions in coronary and cerebrovascular events. In two studies using the fibric acid derivative gemfibrozil, reductions in cardiovascular end points were also achieved.

Lifestyle intervention, including medical nutrition therapy, increased physical activity, weight loss, and smoking cessation, are an important component of therapy. Glycemic control can also beneficially modify plasma lipid levels, particularly in patients with very high triglycerides and poor glycemic control.

It is important to note that clinical trials with fibrates and niacin have demonstrated benefits in patients who were not on treatment with statins and that there are no data available on reduction of events with such

Table 5.16 Lipid management in diabetes

- Test for lipid disorders at least annually and more often if needed to achieve goals.
- Goals: In adults with low-risk lipid values (LDL <100 mg/dL, HDL >50 mg/dL, and triglycerides <150 mg/dL). In individuals with overt CVD: All patients should be treated with a statin to achieve an LDL reduction of 30% to 40%.
- A lower LDL cholesterol goal of <70 mg/dL (1.8 mmol/L), using a high dose of a statin, is an option in high risk patients.
- Lifestyle modification (reduction of saturated fat and cholesterol intake, weight loss and increased physical activity) has been shown to improve the lipid profile in patients with diabetes.
- For those over the age of 40 years, statin therapy to achieve an LDL reduction of 30% to 40% regardless of baseline LDL levels is strongly recommended.
- Lowering triglycerides and increasing HDL cholesterol with a fibrate in patients with diabetic dyslipidemia is associated with a reduction in cardiovascular events in patients with clinical CVD, low HDL, and near-normal levels of LDL, particularly if not treated with a statin.
- Combination therapy using statins and other lipid-lowering agents may be necessary to achieve lipid targets but has not been evaluated in outcomes studies for either CVD event reduction of safety.

Table 5.17 Additional strategies to decrease CVD

Antiplatelet agents
- Aspirin therapy (75 to 32.5 mg/day).
- Combination therapy using other antiplatelet agents such as clopidogrel in addition to aspirin should be used in patients with severe and progressive CVD.
- Aspirin may not be effective for primary prevention.
- Some patients are resistant to Aspirin.

Smoking cessation
- Advise all patients not to smoke.
- Include smoking cessation counseling and other forms of treatment as a routine component of diabetes care.

Other treatments
- ACE inhibitors even in the absence of hypertension or albuminuria.
- β-Blockers for patients with CHD (watch for masking of hypoglycemia symptoms).
- Thiazolidinediones: Pioglitazone has been shown to decrease myocardial infarction, stroke, and death but is associated with fluid retention and the development of congestive heart failure. Caution in prescribing thiazolidinediones in the setting of known congestive heart failure or other heart diseases, as well as in patients with preexisting edema or concurrent insulin therapy, is required.

Reprinted with permission from Fonseca, Pendergrass, and McDuffie. *Handbook of Diabetes*. Current Medicine Group © 2008.

combinations. The risks may be greater in patients who are treated with combinations of these drugs with high doses of statins.

Screening for macrovascular complications

To identify the presence of CHD in diabetic patients without clear or suggestive symptoms of coronary artery disease, a risk factor–based approach to the initial diagnostic evaluation and subsequent follow-up is recommended (see Diabetes PhD at www.diabetes.org or use the Framingham score or UKPDS risk engine).

A diagnostic cardiac stress test should be done in patients with (1) typical or atypical cardiac symptoms and (2) an abnormal resting electrocardiogram (ECG). The screening of asymptomatic patients remains controversial, and a significant proportion of patients may have abnormalities; the significance of this is unclear.[15]

A screening cardiac stress test may be considered (but is not essential) in those with (1) a history of peripheral or carotid occlusive disease and (2) sedentary lifestyle, age >35 years, and plans to begin a vigorous exercise program.

Patients with abnormal exercise ECG and patients unable to perform an exercise ECG require additional or alternative testing. Currently, stress nuclear perfusion and stress echocardiography are valuable next-level diagnostic procedures.

Initial screening for peripheral artery disease should include a history for claudication and an assessment of the pedal pulses. Consider measuring the ankle-brachial pressure index as many patients with peripheral artery disease are asymptomatic, and refer patients with significant or a positive ankle-brachial pressure index for an arterial Doppler study.

Strategy for preventing complications and treating complicated patients

Recent clinical trail data (1–3) has reignited debates about strategies to prevent diabetes complications. As discussed in chapter 1, an aggressive strategy to attempt normoglycemia carries risks, particularly in patients with long standing disease and established complications. On the other hand there is no such risk in patients who are less aggressively managed and they may benefit in terms of at least microvascular complications. The reduction in myocardial infarction using these strategies for intensive treatment was disappointingly not statistically significant. It is unclear whether such interventions will lead to benefits in younger patients with recently diagnosed diabetes and without established complications. The duration of treatment and time to events may also be important. In this context, the UKPDS investigators recently reported the results of the long-term follow-up of patients in the trial, with post-trial monitoring to determine whether this improved glucose control persisted and whether such therapy had a long-term effect on macrovascular outcomes.[18] During the United Kingdom Prospective Diabetes Study (UKPDS), patients with type 2 diabetes mellitus who received intensive glucose therapy had a lower risk of microvascular complications than did those receiving conventional dietary therapy. Of 4209 patients with newly diagnosed type 2 diabetes who were randomly assigned to receive either conventional therapy (dietary restriction) or intensive therapy (either sulfonylurea or insulin or, in overweight patients, metformin) for glucose control, 3277 patients were asked to attend annual UKPDS clinics for five years, but no attempts were made to maintain their previously assigned therapies.[19] Annual questionnaires were used to follow patients who were unable to attend the clinics, and all patients in years 6 to 10 were assessed through questionnaires. Between-group differences in glycated hemoglobin levels were lost after the first year. In the sulfonylurea-insulin group, relative reductions in risk persisted at 10 years for any diabetes-related end point (9%, P = 0.04) and microvascular disease (24%, P = 0.001), and risk reductions for myocardial infarction (15%, P = 0.01) and death from any cause (13%, P = 0.007) emerged over time. In the metformin group, significant risk reductions persisted for any diabetes-related end point (21%, P = 0.01), myocardinal infarction (33%, P = 0.005), and death from any cause (27%, P = 0.002). Thus, despite an early loss of glycemic differences, a continued reduction in microvascular risk and emergent risk reductions for myocardinal infarction and death from any cause were observed during 10 years of post-trial follow-up.[20] A continued benefit after metformin therapy was evident among overweight patients.

References

1. American Diabetes Association. Standards of medical care in diabetes—2007. *Diabetes Care.* 2007;30(suppl 1):S4–S41.

2. Brownlee M. Biochemistry and molecular cell biology of diabetic complications. *Nature.* 2001;414:813–820.

3. Vasudevan AR, Burns A, Fonseca VA. The effectiveness of intensive glycemic control for the prevention of vascular complications in diabetes mellitus. *Treat Endocrinol.* 2006;5:273–286.

4. Stratton IM, Adler AI, Neil HA, et al. Association of glycaemia with macrovascular and microvascular complications of type 2 diabetes (UKPDS 35): prospective observational study. *BMJ.* 2000;321:405–412.

5. ACCORD Study Group, Buse JB, Bigger JT, Byington RP, et al. Action to control cardiovascular risk in diabetes (ACCORD) trial: design and methods. *Am J Cardiol.* 2007;99:21i–33i.

6. Jawa A, Kcomt J, Fonseca VA. Diabetic nephropathy and retinopathy. *Med Clin North Am.* 2004;88:1001, 36, xi.

7. Effect of intensive therapy on the microvascular complications of type 1 diabetes mellitus. *JAMA.* 2002;287:2563–2569.

8. Borch-Johnsen K, Feldt-Rasmussen B, Strandgaard S, Schroll M, Jensen JS. Urinary albumin excretion. An independent predictor of ischemic heart disease. *Arterioscler Thromb Vasc Biol.* 1999;19:1992–1997.

9. Romundstad S, Holmen J, Kvenild K, Hallan H, Ellekjaer H. Microalbuminuria and all-cause mortality in 2,089 apparently healthy individuals: a 4.4-year follow-up study. The Nord-Trondelag Health Study (HUNT), Norway. *Am J Kidney Dis.* 2003;42:466–673.

10. Boulton AJ, Vinik AI, Arezzo JC, et al. Diabetic neuropathies: a statement by the American Diabetes Association. *Diabetes Care.* 2005;28:956–962.

11. Jensen TS, Backonja MM, Hernandez Jimenez S, Tesfaye S, Valensi P, Ziegler D. New perspectives on the management of diabetic peripheral neuropathic pain. *Diab Vasc Dis Res.* 2006;3:108–119.

12. Gaede P, Vedel P, Larsen N, Jensen GV, Parving HH, Pedersen O. Multifactorial intervention and cardiovascular disease in patients with type 2 diabetes. *N Engl J Med.* 2003;348:383–393.

13. Gaede P, Lund-Andersen H, Parving HH, Pedersen O. Effect of a multifactorial intervention on mortality in type 2 diabetes. *N Engl J Med.* 2008;358:580–591.

14. Fonseca V, Desouza C, Asnani S, Jialal I. Nontraditional risk factors for cardiovascular disease in diabetes. *Endocr Rev.* 2004;25:153–175.

15. Wackers FJ, Young LH, Inzucchi SE, et al. Detection of silent myocardial ischemia in asymptomatic diabetic subjects: the DIAD study. *Diabetes Care.* 2004;27:1954–1961.

16. UK Prospective Diabetes Study (UKPDS) Group. Intensive blood-glucose control with sulphonylureas or insulin compared with conventional treatment and risk of complications in patients with type 2 diabetes (UKPDS 33). *Lancet.* 1998;352:837–853.

17. Ohkubo Y, Kishikawa H, Araki E, et al. Intensive insulin therapy prevents the progression of diabetic microvascular complications in Japanese patients with non-insulin-dependent diabetes mellitus: a randomized prospective 6-year study. *Diabetes Res Clin Pract.* 1995;28:103–117.

18. Action to Control Cardiovascular Risk in Diabetes Study Group, Gerstein HC, Miller ME, et al. Effects of instensive glucoselowering 2 diabetes. *N Engl J Med.* 2008;358:2545–2559.

19. The ADVANCE Collaborative Group. Intensive blood glucose control and vascular outcomes in patients with type 2 diabetes. *N Engl J Med.* 2008; 358:2560–2572.

20. Holman RR, Paul SK, Bethel MA, Neil HA, Matthews DR. Long-term follow-up after tight control of blood glucose pressure in type 2 diabetes. *N Engl J Med.* 2008;359:1565–1576.

Chapter 6

Facilitating motivation for self-care in patients with diabetes

Richard R. Rubin and Mark Peyrot

The opportunity

Research has clearly demonstrated that reducing hyperglycemia, blood pressure, and lipids through medication and healthy living can reduce diabetes progression and cardiovascular risk. For example, the Diabetes Control and Complications Trial (DCCT) demonstrated that intensive diabetes treatment improved microvascular and macrovascular outcomes in patients with type 1 diabetes.[1,2] The U.K. Prospective Diabetes Study (UKPDS) found similar benefits of intensive treatment in patients with type 2 diabetes.[3]

Recently, the Look AHEAD trial has convincingly shown that patients with type 2 diabetes can lose weight through an intervention designed to decrease caloric intake and increase activity. Participants in the Look AHEAD active lifestyle intervention lost an average of 8.6 lb during their first year in the study, compared with an average weight loss of 0.7 lb in the diabetes education control intervention. Look AHEAD active lifestyle intervention participants also had significantly greater improvements than control arm participants in a variety of cardiovascular risk factors, including Hb_{A1c}, fitness, systolic and diastolic blood pressure, triglycerides, HDL cholesterol, and urine-to-creatinine ratio.[4]

These studies have included large samples of individuals who were able to adhere to lifestyle change and medication protocols incorporated into these clinical trials so that effects of these interventions could be adequately documented.

The problem

Applying the results of these (and other) landmark studies to the world of clinical practice has been more difficult than expected. Data from the National Health and Nutrition Examination Surveys (NHANES) show that fewer than half of all patients with diabetes reach target-level goals for each of the three key factors that affect long-term diabetes outcomes

(Hb$_{A1c}$ level, blood pressure, and cholesterol level) and that fewer than 10% of these patients reach all three target goals.[5] One important reason for this relative lack of success in achieving risk factor control is low levels of adherence to treatment recommendations by patients with diabetes.

Data from the Diabetes Attitudes Wishes and Needs (DAWN) study of almost 4000 physicians and nurses from 13 countries showed that these health care providers believed that the vast majority of their patients with diabetes did not follow treatment recommendations. According to this survey, only about 7% of patients with type 1 diabetes and 2% of patients with type 2 diabetes completely followed most treatment recommendations. Among the more than 5000 patients participating in the DAWN study, estimates of regimen adherence were somewhat higher—just over 30% for patients with each type of diabetes (Figure 6.1).[6]

So it is possible for patients to manage their diabetes in ways that dramatically improve their chances for a longer, healthier life, but few patients actually do so.

The heart of the matter

It is not surprising that in clinical practice, at national meetings, and in the literature, the two related questions voiced most often by practicing clinicians are:

- How do I help my patients take better care of their diabetes?
- How do I do this in the limited time I have with them?

We reviewed the literature addressing these issues in a recent review.[7] The current chapter focuses on practical applications of the review.

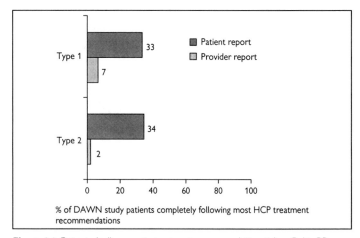

Figure 6.1 Estimated adherence to treatment recommendations is low. Rubin RR, Peyrot M. Patients' and providers' perspectives on diabetes care: results of the Diabetes Attitudes, Wishes, and Needs (DAWN) study. *Practical Diabetology*. 2005;24:6–13.

Patient motivation is the key to success

The vast majority of diabetes care is self-care. Countless times each day patients make clinically relevant decisions (every time they decide what to eat, when to eat, how much to eat; when to exercise, how much to exercise, how intensively to exercise; when to take medication, which medication to take, how much medication to take; when to monitor blood glucose, how frequently to monitor; when to call clinician). So the patient is truly the primary provider of diabetes care.

Thus the clinician's primary roles must be those of advisor, facilitator, and coach. This is very different from the role most clinicians were trained to assume, and very different from their appropriate role in treating acute conditions; it is, however, the only effective role clinicians can play in treating a chronic condition such as diabetes where success depends primarily on effective self-care.

Patient motivation is the key to active self-care, but many are not clear on what motivation actually is. Motivation is an internal state. As we will attempt to demonstrate in this chapter, sources of motivation are personal and multidetermined and may be unique to the individual. We also will discuss the fact that people are often not fully conscious of the sources of their motivation. Clinicians can help patients uncover these sources of their motivation through the application of relatively straightforward practical techniques.

Facilitating motivation is feasible in clinical practice

To be useful in clinical practice, an approach must be feasible—it must respect the limited time clinicians have with their patients and the fact that most clinicians are not trained in facilitating motivation. Interventions we discuss respect these limits; they incorporate the following concepts:

- Simplicity
- Ease of application
- Use of other providers and other resources
- Suggestions for step-by-step, visit-by-visit approach; not everything can be done in one visit, and it does not need to be

We also note the consequences of not using the approaches we recommend, including "spinning wheels" visit after visit, making no progress in efforts to help patients improve self-care, and consequent poor clinical outcomes. The approaches we recommend have an additional benefit; they improve patient and clinician morale and well-being.

Facilitating motivation: Key steps

To effectively facilitate patient motivation for diabetes self-care, the clinician must do the following:

- **ENGAGE** the patient
- **EVALUATE** the patient's knowledge, health literacy, self-care behavior, financial resources, and emotional well-being

- **ELUCIDATE** the patient's self-care goals
- **ENCOURAGE** the patient's efforts to reach self-care goals

In the remainder of this chapter, we offer suggestions for success with each of these steps.

ENGAGE *the patient*

The first step in facilitating motivation for diabetes self-care is engaging the patient, and the *sine qua non* of engaging the patient is helping him or her identify personally meaningful diabetes-related concerns. We must recognize that people are motivated *only* by concerns or problems that are personally meaningful. When patients identify problems that trouble them, it is better to start with those problems, unless the clinician has identified an issue that is immediately life-threatening or debilitating.

This approach has several advantages; because patients are more likely to work hard to resolve personally meaningful problems, they are more likely to succeed in addressing those problems, and this increases patients' confidence in their own ability to change. In addition, when the clinician helps patients identify and resolve personally meaningful problems, it increases the clinician's credibility and thus his or her influence, strengthening the therapeutic relationship.

The key to identifying concerns that will motivate change is asking good questions. Good questions are open-ended—for example:

- "What is the hardest thing for you right now about living with diabetes?"
- "What do we need to talk about today?"

Good questions help the patient identify a "sticking point"—a problem that is defined as specifically as possible, because the more specific the problem, the easier it is to address it effectively. For example, a problem of "I can't stop snacking after dinner" is easier to address than "I can't stick to my diet." With thoughtful questioning (e.g., "You say you can't stick to your diet; could you be more specific about when you have the hardest time?"), any patient can identify one or more specific sticking points. We recommend asking patients to identify a personally meaningful problem specifically enough for the clinician to be able to picture it. It is difficult to picture "I can't stick to my diet"; it is much easier to picture "I can't stop snacking after dinner."

Identifying specific patient "sticking points" has several benefits. First, it helps protect patients from the tendency to "catastrophize," to feel that they are doing everything wrong, by making it clear that the most serious problems ("sticking points") are fairly confined. We find that most patients are relieved to discover their sticking points. In addition, identifying a sticking point provides a specific focus for efforts to improve self-care and well-being, and this can dramatically improve efficiency and effectiveness of patient–provider interactions. Finally, identifying sticking points provides relief for the clinician, who may feel as overwhelmed as the patient when faced with broad, ill-defined problems and very limited time.

EVALUATE *the patient's knowledge, health literacy, self-care behavior, financial resources, and emotional well-being*

Knowledge

Patients cannot manage their diabetes well unless they understand their disease and what it takes to maintain good health, so patient knowledge must be assessed through direct questions. To be clear, knowledge alone is not sufficient for optimal diabetes self-care, because self-care skill and emotional coping skills are also essential, but without knowledge good self-care is impossible. Again, open-ended questions are most effective for evaluating knowledge. Here are two examples:

- "Do you feel that you know enough to manage your diabetes effectively?"
- "If the answer is no, what additional information do you need?"

These questions can be asked by the clinician or by office staff, including nurses, dietitians, or nursing assistants, if they are available. Structured questionnaires such as the Michigan Diabetes Research and Training Center Brief Diabetes Knowledge Test[8] can also be used to assess knowledge. Patients who need diabetes education should be provided the information they need by the clinician, by office staff, or by referral to a diabetes educator.

Health literacy

Almost half of adults in the United States have inadequate health literacy—they cannot understand basic medical advice. Unfortunately, inadequate health literacy frequently goes unrecognized because clinicians rarely verify that patients understand what they have been told. As a consequence, patients are often incapable of following treatment recommendations. Patients with diabetes who have inadequate health literacy have higher Hb_{A1c} levels, controlling for other factors that might be associated with glycemic control.[9]

Clinicians can assess patients' health literacy by asking one simple question: "How often do you have difficulty understanding written medical information?" Any response other than "never" strongly suggests that the patient has health literacy problems.

Clinicians can minimize health literacy problems and help patients understand medical advice by avoiding jargon. Studies show that even words and terms that seem easy to understand (e.g., *stable*, *more frequently*) often are not understood. Other studies demonstrate that the use of jargon is very common and that verifying patient comprehension is rare. In one study of interactions between clinicians and patients with diabetes, physicians assessed recall and comprehension only 12% of the time when new concepts were presented.[10] Often, these new concepts involved critical issues such as adjustment of medication. It is very important to note that visits including assessment of recall and comprehension were no longer than those that did not include this assessment. Using the teach-back method is the key to ensuring patient recall and comprehension. As we just pointed out, this approach need not add time to visits. Here are the steps in the teach-back method:

- Explain (e.g., "You will be taking this new medication, called metformin, before breakfast and dinner. You will be taking one pill before each of these meals.")
- Assess (e.g., "To be sure I explained clearly, please tell me what you heard")
- Clarify (if assessment reveals any misunderstanding; offer support in the form of written instructions if necessary)
- Reassess (if patient misunderstood original instructions). Patient understands and is able to recall instructions (Figure 6.2)

Self-care

As noted at the beginning of this chapter, adherence to diabetes self-care recommendations is often limited. Clinicians can assess self-care behavior by asking two simple questions:

- "How closely do you follow recommendations for healthy eating, exercise, blood glucose monitoring, and taking medications?"
- "What self-care skills would you like to improve?"

Patients who need and want to improve self-care practices should be provided the skill-based education they require from the clinician, from office staff, or from a diabetes educator.

Resources

The typical patient with diabetes takes an average of nine different medications each day, and many patients with diabetes do not take prescribed medication due to cost. Research shows that many patients do not tell their clinicians that they are not taking their prescribed medication, and the most common reason given for not telling is that the clinician never asked.[11] Even when a clinician does ask about medication adherence, the issue of cost as a barrier to adherence is rarely raised.

Clinicians can assess this issue by asking two simple questions:

- "Will the cost of this medication be a problem for you?"
- "Since your last visit, have you ever taken less of your medication than prescribed because of the cost?"

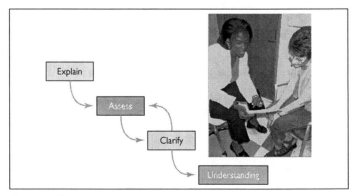

Figure 6.2 Teach-back method.

When cost is a barrier to medication adherence, the clinician can address the issue in an appropriate manner—by adjusting prescriptions or by helping the patient find sources of support to pay for the medication.

Emotional well-being

The Diabetes Attitudes, Wishes, and Needs (DAWN) study surveyed over 4000 clinicians who treated patients with diabetes from 13 countries. More than three-fourths of these clinicians said psychological problems (disorders or high levels of diabetes-related distress) interfered with their patients' ability to follow treatment recommendations.[2]

Depression is the most common psychological disorder in patients with diabetes; major depressive disorder, the most serious form of clinical depression, is 1.5 to 2 times as common among people with diabetes as it is in the general population, and significant symptoms of depression are at least twice as common among people with diabetes as they are in the general population.[12,13]

Depression among patients with diabetes is associated with less active self-care and with higher levels of Hb_{A1c}, complications, mortality, and health care expenditures as well. It is important to note that even relatively low levels of depression symptoms are associated with these negative clinical outcomes,[14] so it is important to identify patients who might be depressed.

Clinicians can identify patients who might be suffering from depression by asking two simple questions that address the two cardinal symptoms of depression. These questions are presented in Table 6.1.

Patients who might be depressed can be referred to a mental health professional for a definitive diagnosis and treatment. The clinician might also choose to treat the patient for depression without referral.

Depression in patients with diabetes can be effectively treated by medication or counseling, and effective depression treatment is associated with improved glucose control in patients with high glucose levels prior to depression treatment. Patients with depression are likely to experience relapse and should be monitored closely to determine if this occurs.

Table 6.1 Questions to identify patients who might be depressed
• Over the last 2 weeks, how often have you been bothered by little interest or pleasure in doing things?
• not at all [0]
• several days [1]
• more than half the days [2]
• nearly every day [3]
• Over the last 2 weeks, how often have you been bothered by feeling down, depressed, or hopeless?
• not at all [0]
• several days [1]
• more than half the days [2]

Diabetes distress

Diabetes-related distress is associated with less active self-care and many of the same consequent negative clinical outcomes associated with depression. Patients sometimes spontaneously express this distress, often in terms of feeling demoralized about their ability to manage their diabetes. Patients who might be distressed can be identified by asking questions such as the following, designed to assess specific sources of distress:

• "Do you feel overwhelmed by the demands of living with diabetes?"
• "Do family and friends give you the emotional support you need?"
• "Do you think you will end up with diabetes complications no matter what you do?"

Diabetes distress can also be assessed using the validated Diabetes Distress Scale (DDS).[15]

Helping patients recognize the power of "self-talk" (what they say to themselves) can provide relief from diabetes-related distress. This is the foundation of cognitive-behavioral therapy (CBT), which is also an effective treatment for depression and which is readily available from mental health specialists. CBT is designed to help people identify negative, usually unrealistic thoughts that lead to distress, diminished motivation, and less active self-care (e.g., "I'll never be able to do anything right"). CBT also helps patients find more positive, realistic perspectives on diabetes-related problems and practice and apply the new perspective, thus relieving distress, enhancing motivation, and encouraging more active self-care. The principles of CBT are straightforward, and clinicians can incorporate strategies based on these principles into their work with patients.[16]

ELUCIDATING *an action plan*

Research has shown that intentions are major determinants of self-care behavior. Goal setting, a procedure for translating patients' behavior change intentions into goals, is essential to establishing and maintaining an effective diabetes self-care plan. Goals that are set should be "SMART":

• **S**pecific: based on concrete actions (e.g., not snacking after dinner) rather than values (e.g., healthy eating)
• **M**easurable: how much, how often (e.g., walk 30 minutes three times a week)
• **A**ction oriented: address behavior (e.g., exercise) rather than physiology (e.g., losing weight)
• **R**ealistic but challenging: not so difficult that patients become discouraged or so easy to reach that they provide no sense of accomplishment
• **T**ime-based, timely, tangible, trackable

Table 6.2 illustrates steps in the process of action planning or goal setting.

This process can be effective with a patient who is interested in making changes to improve diabetes self-care.

Table 6.2 Elucidating a diabetes action plan

Step 1:	Identify a personally meaningful issue.
Step 2:	Assess current behavior.
Step 3:	Focus on *behavior* change.
Step 4:	Set a specific goal.
Step 5:	Be sure the goal is realistic.
Step 6:	Pin down the details.
Step 7:	Prepare for pitfalls.
Step 8:	Close the deal.

- **Step One: Identify a Personally Meaningful Issue**

  Clinician: "What bothers you most right now about your diabetes?"

  Patient: "I'm worried about diabetes complications, like problems with my eyes or my kidneys."

- **Step Two: Assess Current Behavior**

  Clinician: "What are you doing right now to protect yourself from those problems?"

  Patient: "Not as much as I should. I just have to get my blood sugars down where they belong."

- **Step Three: Focus on Behavior Change**

  Clinician: "What are you thinking of?"

  Patient: "Everybody tells me I need to eat healthier, but that's so tough for me. I used to be really good about walking, but then I let it slide."

- **Step Four: Set Specific Goal**

  Clinician: "That could help. How often and how far will you walk?"

  Patient: "I used to walk an hour each day, but I'm not in great shape now, so maybe half an hour a day."

- **Step Five: Be Sure the Goal Is Realistic**

  Clinician: "Sounds like you were a serious walker! Does even half an hour every day sound realistic to you?"

  Patient: "I guess you are right; I could start with 5 days a week."

- **Step Six: Pin Down the Details**

  Clinician: "When will you walk?"

  Patient: "I'll try Saturday and Sunday morning, and Tuesday, Wednesday and Thursday after dinner."

- **Step Seven: Prepare for Pitfalls**

  Clinician: "Can you think of anything that could keep you from walking this Saturday?"

  Patient: "If I stay up too late watching DVD movies the night before."

- **Step Eight: Close the Deal**

Clinician: "Let me sure I have your plan straight. You will watch only one DVD tomorrow night, walk 30 minutes Saturday and Sunday morning, and 3 days during the week."

Patient: "That's right."

Clinician: "May I check with you in 2 weeks to see how things are going?"

Patient: "Sure."

ENCOURAGE *patients to reach their goals*

Once patients have identified self-care goals, they need encouragement to reach these goals. Here we offer suggestions for effective approaches to encouragement (Table 6.3).

Encourage patients to keep their eyes on the prize

Slipping from active self-care efforts is almost inevitable unless there is a very good reason not to, so clinicians can facilitate ongoing self-care by helping patients identify a personally meaningful reason for working so hard to manage their diabetes. Identifying this reason and keeping it in mind is a key to maintaining motivation for active self-care. Clinicians can ask patients directly to identify their personal reason for working hard to manage their diabetes. We have found that the most effective reasons are both personal and positive. Personally meaningful motivators may be unique to the individual, but they often have to do with continuing to enjoy family, friends, and favorite activities.

Encourage patients to look for lessons

No one manages diabetes perfectly; the only way anyone learns is through trial and error. We have found that it often helps patients to think of their self-care efforts, includng those that were unsuccessful, as experiments. This can help to minimize the distress associated with diabetes-related mistakes, and it helps patients focus on what they might do differently next time, based on the consequences of the mistake. Ask patients to identify a recent diabetes-related experiment/mistake, and what lesson they could draw from it.

Encourage patients to focus on what went right

It is natural for clinicians and patients to focus on self-care mistakes or lapses, in an effort to correct those mistakes, but there is great benefit in

Table 6.3 Encouraging patients to reach their self-care goals

Encourage patients to:
- Keep their eyes on the prize
- Look for lessons
- Focus on what went right
- Draw on others
- Reward themselves for reaching self-care goals
- Look on the light side
- Prevent a lapse from becoming a relapse

focusing on what went right rather than what went wrong. Focusing on what went right improves the perspective of both clinician and patient. Focusing on what went right makes it clear that *some* things did go right, minimizing feelings of discouragement and hopelessness. Even more important, focusing on what went right allows the clinician and patient to identify *why* things went right when they did, thus increasing the likelihood that things will go right more often in the future. Ask patients about a recent self-care success, what contributed to the success, and what lesson they could learn from that success.

Encourage patients to draw on others
Daily life with diabetes is demanding, so most patients need to draw on others to be successful. Some patients need more support than others. Some patients need practical support, some need emotional support, and some need both. Ask patients the following questions to help them get the support they need from family and friends:
- *"What do your family and friends do that makes it easier to manage your diabetes?"*
- *"What do they do that makes it harder?"*
- *"What could they (realistically) do to make things easier?"*

Encourage patients to ask for the support they need. Ask patients what *you* can do to help make their lives with diabetes easier.

Encourage patients to reward themselves for reaching self-care goals
Rewards for reaching self-care goals can help maintain motivation for the hard work of diabetes self-management. Clinicians can help patients identify personally meaningful rewards, from the ethereal (e.g., feeling you are a better person) to the material (e.g., that new dress you really want). Rewards and the criteria for receiving them should be clear. Ask patients about personally meaningful rewards for reaching self-care goals.

Encourage patients to look on the light side
Laughter is a great stress reliever ("I don't know how I would have made it if it weren't for my sense of humor" is something we often hear). Relieving stress reduces anxiety and makes problem solving and goal attainment easier. For better and for worse, diabetes gives patients lots to laugh at, if they take the right perspective. Ask patients about any humorous diabetes-related experiences they have had. Most patients we know have had such experiences. Clinicians can also collect humorous diabetes-related stories to share with patients who are interested in hearing them

Encourage patients to prevent a lapse from becoming a relapse
Occasional lapses in self-care are almost impossible to avoid, because it is easier for people to eat whatever they want and to not exercise or monitor blood glucose than to do what is required to actively manage diabetes. So your patients' goal should be avoiding as many lapses as they can and preventing full-blown relapses. When patients are tempted to lapse they may be able to resist the temptation if they are feeling strong and confident, and if they can keep in mind their personal reason(s) for working so hard to manage their diabetes.

Sometimes patients who do lapse recognize what is happening and find the strength and confidence to get back on track. Ask patients questions to help them identify things that put them at risk for a lapse; these may include internal urges (e.g., feeling like celebrating with extra food), negative emotions (e.g., feeling angry, lonely, bored), something bad happening (e.g., accident, money worries), stress with another person (e.g., an argument), or social pressure (e.g., people encouraging unhealthy eating).

Help patients identify ways to protect themselves from a lapse or relapse; these may include avoiding situations that trigger lapses, recognizing tricks their minds play (e.g., "I've had a really hard day; I deserve that extra dessert"), remembering that a lapse is not a relapse (e.g., stay calm, recognize that a lapse is natural and inevitable, and that getting back on track and avoiding a relapse is possible), and keeping one's personal motivator in mind (e.g., "I want to be around to see my grandson get his high school diploma"). Ask patients where they will turn for help to prevent a lapse from becoming a relapse.

Summary and conclusions

Controlling blood glucose, blood pressure, and cholesterol levels is the key to living a longer, healthier life with diabetes, yet very few patients reach accepted targets for all of these three factors. Because self-care represents the vast majority of diabetes care, facilitating self-care is a *sine qua non* of improved diabetes outcomes. Unfortunately, few clinicians have been extensively trained in facilitating self-care, and this kind of facilitation is very different from the most effective approaches to treating acute conditions.

To effectively facilitate diabetes self-care, clinicians must (1) **ENGAGE** the patient; (2) **EVAUATE** self-care knowledge, health literacy, financial barriers to treatment adherence, and emotional well-being; (3) **ELUCIDATE** a self-care action plan; and (4) **ENCOURAGE** patients in their efforts to reach self-care goals. In this chapter we have provided suggestions for accomplishing these objectives. We have focused on recommendations that are simple, are effective, and do not take much time. We hope that these recommendations help you facilitate self-care in your patients who have diabetes, thus improving clinical outcomes and the satisfaction you and your patients find in your work together.

References

1. The Diabetes Control and Complications Trial Research Group. The effect of intensive treatment of diabetes on the development and progression of long-term complications in insulin-dependent diabetes mellitus. *N Engl J Med.* 1993;329:977–986.

2. The Diabetes Control and Complications Trial/Epidemiology of Diabetes Interventions and Complications (DCCT/EDICT) Study Research Group. Intensive diabetes treatment and cardiovascular disease in patients with type 1 diabetes. *N Engl J Med.* 2005;353:2643–2653.

3. UK Prospective Diabetes Study (UKPDS) Group. Intensive blood glucose control with sulfonylureas compared with conventional treatment and risk of complications in patients with type 2 diabetes. *Lancet.* 1998;352:837–853.

4. The Look AHEAD Research Group. Reduction in weight and cardiovascular disease risk factors in individuals with type 2 diabetes: one-year results of the Look AHEAD Trial. *Diabetes Care.* 2007;30:1374–1383.

5. Saydah SH, Fradkin J, Cowie CC. Poor control of risk factors for vascular disease among adults with previously diagnosed diabetes. *JAMA.* 2004;291:335–342.

6. Rubin RR, Peyrot M. Patients' and providers' perspectives on diabetes care: results of the Diabetes Attitudes, Wishes, and Needs (DAWN) Study. *Pract Diabetol.* 2005;24:6–13.

7. Peyrot M, Rubin RR. Behavioral and psychosocial interventions in diabetes: a conceptual review. *Diabetes Care.* 2007;30:2433–2440.

8. Fitzgerald JT, Funnell MM, Hess GE, et al. The reliability and validity of a brief diabetes knowledge test. *Diabetes Care.* 1998;21:706–710.

9. Schillinger D, Grumbach K, Piette J, et al. Association of health literacy with diabetes outcomes. *JAMA.* 2002;288:475–482.

10. Schillinger D, Piette J, Grumbach K, et al. Closing the loop: physician communication with diabetic patients who have low health literacy. *Arch Intern Med.* 2003;163:83–90.

11. Piette J, Heisler M, Wagner TH. Cost-related medication underuse: do patients with chronic illnesses tell their doctors? *Arch Intern Med.* 2004;164:1749–1755.

12. Egede LE, Zheng D. Independent factors associated with major depressive disorder in a national sample. *Diabetes Care.* 2003;26:104–111.

13. Anderson RJ, Freedland KE, Clouse RE, Lustman PJ. The prevalence of comorbid depression in adults with diabetes. *Diabetes Care.* 2001;24:1069–1078.

14. Black SA, Markides KS, Ray LA. Depression predicts increased incidence of adverse health outcomes in older Mexican Americans with type 2 diabetes. *Diabetes Care.* 2003;26:2822–2828.

15. Polonsjy WH, Fisher L, Earles J, et al. Assessing psychosocial distress in diabetes: development of the Diabetes Distress Scale. *Diabetes Care.* 2005;28:626–631.

16. Rollnick S, Mason P, Butler B. *Health Behavior Change: A Guide for Practitioners.* London: Churchill Livingstone; 1999.

Chapter 7

Diet recommendations and patient education

Susie Wiegert Villalobos

For people living with diabetes, diet and self-care skills form the foundation of good diabetes control. The progressive nature and ever-expanding knowledge base of diabetes care require that patient education be an ongoing process between the patient and his or her health care team. Education goals must be based on the abilities of the patient and the treatment plan the physician has outlined and be tailored to fit the individual needs of each patient. The American Diabetes Association (ADA), in conjunction with the American Association of Diabetes Educators, the American Dietetic Association, the Veterans Health Administration, the Centers for Disease Control and Prevention, the Indian Health service, and the American Pharmaceutical Association, has worked toward establishing national standards for diabetes self-management education. These standards guide the organization and lend structure to any education program that is approved by the ADA to have the designation as a "Recognized Education Program."

Tables 7.1 through 7.4 outline key factors that should be addressed with all patients with diabetes.

Diabetes, a chronic and progressive disease, can have highly variable patient health outcomes. How well patients are managed is heavily affected by the degree to which a patient practices diabetes-related self-care behaviors. Ideally, the patient's treatment plan and education goals are revised and adapted throughout the years according to individual patient needs.

An integral part of the diabetes education process involves diet and, specifically, how food choices influence the overall health and well-being of a diabetic patient. As will be outlined later in this chapter, there are many "meal planning" methods to improve blood glucose levels and other comorbid conditions influenced by diet. The role of the registered dietitian is to help each patient find a plan that will best serve his or her needs and abilities to obtain improved health and diabetes control.

Medical nutrition therapy (MNT) is the "nutritional diagnostic, therapy, and counseling services for the purpose of disease management which are furnished by a registered dietitian or nutrition professional for the purpose of managing a disease."[3] MNT and meal planning form the foundation of blood sugar control; without proper attention paid to food consumption, a patient's medical treatment plan will ultimately fail.

Table 7.1 Patient education

- An individual education assessment should be performed for each patient to assess educational needs.
- A plan should be outlined to accomplish goals dictated by patient needs.
- Follow-up appointments should be scheduled PRN.
- Outpatient education
  - Comprehensive diabetes self-management education (see Core Curriculum for DSME)
- In-patient education
  - Survival skills only (meal plan, hypoglycemia/hyperglycemia, urine ketone testing [if applicable], blood glucose monitoring, medication, obtaining diabetic supplies, sick day management)
  - Follow-up outpatient appointments usually necessary

Table 7.2 The AADE7 self-care behaviors[1]

- Healthy eating
- Being active
- Monitoring
- Taking medication
- Problem solving
- Healthy coping
- Reducing risks

Source: American Association of Diabetes Educators. Definitions; AADE 7™ Self-care Behaviors. Available at: http://www.diabeteseducator.org/ProfessionalResources/AADE7. Accessed April 24, 2008.

Table 7.3 Core curriculum for diabetes self-management education (DSME)[2]

- Describing the diabetes disease process and treatment options
- Incorporating nutritional management into lifestyle
- Incorporating physical activity into lifestyle
- Using medication(s) safely and for maximum therapeutic effectiveness
- Monitoring blood glucose and other parameters and interpreting and using the results for self-management decision making
- Preventing, detecting, and treating acute complications
- Preventing detecting, and treating chronic complications
- Developing personal strategies to address psychosocial issues and concerns
- Developing personal strategies to promote health and behavior change

Source: Funnell M, Brown TL, Childs BP, et al. National standards for diabetes self-management education. *Diabetes Care.* 2007;30:1632.

Table 7.4 Seven principles for controlling your diabetes for life[4]

1. Learn as much as you can about diabetes.
2. Get regular care for your diabetes.
3. Learn how to manage your diabetes.
4. Control the ABCs of diabetes (A1c, Blood pressure, Cholesterol).
5. Monitor your diabetes ABCs.
6. Prevent long-term diabetes problems.
7. Get checked for long-term problems and treat them.

Source: American Dietetic Association. Definitions in the Medicare MNT benefit proposed regulations: medical nutrition therapy. Available at: http://www.eatright.org/cps/rde/xchg/ada/hs.xsl/nutrition_3391_ENU_HTML.htm. Accessed April 24, 2008.

Table 7.5 MNT goals for people with diabetes[5]

1. Achieve and maintain:
   • blood glucose levels as close to normal as safely possible.
   • lipid and lipoprotein profile that reduces the risk for vascular disease.
   • blood pressure levels in the normal range or as close to normal as is safely possible.
2. To prevent, or at least slow, the rate of development of the chronic complications of diabetes by modifying nutrient intake and lifestyle.
3. To address individual nutrition needs, taking into account personal and cultural preferences and willingness to change.
4. To maintain the pleasure of eating by only eliminating food choices when indicated by scientific evidence.

Source: American Diabetes Association. Nutrition recommendations and interventions for diabetes. A position statement of the American Diabetes Association. *Diabetes Care*. 2008;31(suppl 1):S61.

Usually, several sessions with a registered dietitian are necessary to ensure a good understanding of meal planning principles. Progress in meal planning is highly dependent on the patient's level of interest, intellectual capability, and education level. Follow-up sessions are usually scheduled as needed or when indicated by a change in treatment plan, such as going from non-hypoglycemia-causing oral medications to hypoglycemia-causing oral medications and/or insulin.

The first step in the nutrition care process is a nutrition assessment, which involves evaluating objective and subjective data collected about a patient's usual food and supplement intake, lifestyle, and past medical history. The health care provider can then evaluate a patient's nutritional deficits and create a treatment plan to help the patient reach a better state of health. The necessary components of a complete assessment include anthropometric measurements, biochemical data, clinical observations, and patient medical history. This list includes but is not limited to height, weight, goal weight, physical activity level, and, of course, disease state. All of these important health markers will help guide a practitioner toward a desirable calorie and macronutrient and micronutrient range for the patient.

Table 7.6 Nutrition assessment components

- Anthropometric measurements
  - Height
  - Weight (actual, usual, and ideal or desirable body weight)
  - Body mass index (BMI)
- Biochemical markers
  - Lab values with nutritional implications
    - Albumin
    - Glucose
    - Lipids
    - Hb_{A1c}
    - BUN
    - Cr
    - GFR
    - Hemoglobin and hematocrit
- Clinical observations
- Patient medical history (includes diet history)
- Medical and surgical
- Medication and supplements
- Diet
- Family

Guidelines for assessing/calculating calorie requirements

There are several methods for estimating the caloric needs of patients. Some methods are better suited to certain populations than others.

Children

- Children's physical measurements should be plotted on growth charts to determine height/weight adequacy.
- If a child's height and weight are within normal limits, use actual body weight.
- If a child is determined to be "at risk for overweight" (body mass index [BMI] between 85th and 95th percentiles) or "overweight" (95th percentile or greater), then expected body weight (EBW) or height should be used to determine caloric needs.

(kcal/kg) RDA energy
- Age 0 to 3 = ≈100
- 4 to 6 = ≈90
- 7 to 10 = ≈70

Females
- 11 to 14 = ≈47
- 15 to 18 = ≈40
- 19 to 24 = ≈38 (may be considered "adult")

Males
- 11 to 14 = ≈55
- 15 to 18 = ≈45
- 19 to 24 = ≈40 (may be considered "adult")

Adults
- Determine ideal or desirable body weight.
- If patient's weight is less than the ideal, use actual body weight.

Adults, Male

5 ft 0 in = 106 lb, then 6 lb for each additional inch
(±10% depending on body frame size)

kcal/kg

Age >25 = ≈30 to 35
If overweight to obese, for very sedentary patients, or for the elderly
= ≈20 to 25

Adults, Female

5 ft 0 in = 100 lb, then 5 lb for each additional inch (±10% depending on body frame size)

Pregnancy
- Use above guidelines, but add 300 calories for the second and third trimester.

Meal planning

In general, patients with diabetes will follow or learn about the Diabetic Exchange List, a constant carbohydrate meal plan or carbohydrate counting to help control his or her blood sugar level. Usually, the registered dietitian (RD) will select a meal plan on a patient-by-patient basis. The RD may combine several methods or may start with one plan and change to another based on patient needs. Regardless of which meal planning method is chosen, counseling sessions should be individualized.

Table 7.7 Meal plan options
• Diabetic exchange lists
• Constant carbohydrate meal plan
• Carbohydrate counting
• Simplified meal plans (plate method)

Diabetic Exchange List

The foundation for most patients is to start with the Diabetic Exchange List, because it is a relatively easy way to categorize "like" foods into one of six groups (starch, fruit, milk, nonstarchy vegetables, protein, and fat). Foods within a given group have similar macronutrient compositions based on serving sizes. Mastery of these food groups allows patients to estimate carbohydrate intake via predetermined portions. Patients are assigned a daily food/meal exchange (e.g., breakfast: 2 starches, 1 fruit, 1 protein, and 1 fat). Once the meal plan has been determined, foods can be "exchanged" within a group without compromising the macronutrient (carbohydrate, protein, and fat) mix. Some patients find this method too restrictive for long-term adherence.

Constant carbohydrate meal plan

An alternative method is the constant carbohydrate meal plan. This plan entails eating a set amount of carbohydrate at a given meal/snack. The "type" or "group" of carbohydrate is not emphasized; instead the amount of carbohydrate (grams of carbohydrate) becomes the focus. This can be particularly useful either for patients not on any medicine or for those on fixed-dose insulin regimens or oral medications taken at set times. This method offers more freedom than the exchange system in that the patient gets to choose what type of carbohydrate he or she would like to consume, but it does not allow any variation in the quantity of carbohydrate. Most patients start with learning the exchange system to learn 15 g carbohydrate portions.

Carbohydrate counting method

The carbohydrate counting method offers the patient a great deal of flexibility compared to the previously mentioned methods. In this method, the patient varies his or her insulin dose to match the amount of carbohydrate he or she will consume. Carbohydrate counting is more advanced and assumes that the patient has a very good working knowledge of the

Table 7.8 Diabetic exchange list (key points)

- Food divided into six groups:
  - starch, milk, fruit, nonstarchy vegetables, protein, fat
- Foods within a group have similar macronutrient compositions based on serving sizes.
- Foods within groups can be "exchanged" with one another.
- Some patients find this method too restrictive for long-term adherence.

Table 7.9 Constant carbohydrate meal plan (key points)

- Set amount of carbohydrate for meals and snacks.
- Patient chooses what type of carbohydrate; only concern is total grams of carbohydrate.
- Flexible meal choices, but not flexible in quantity.

Table 7.10 Carbohydrate counting method (key points)

- Patient uses carbohydrate (CHO)-to-insulin ratio (CIR) to determine how much rapid-acting insulin to dose based on how much CHO she or he plans on eating.
- May not be appropriate for all patients
  - Requires good portion size estimation skills and some basic math skills.
- For example, 1:15 CIR; meal 60 g CHO ÷ 15 = 4 units rapid-acting insulin
  - If preprandial and postprandial blood glucose (BG) levels are close to the same number, dose and estimate of CHO were correct.
  - If postprandial BG ↑, not enough rapid-acting insulin was taken (patient may have underestimated CHO portion).
  - If postprandial BG ↓, too much rapid-acting insulin was taken (patient may have overestimated CHO portion).
  - If BG is ↑ or ↓ for all values, the basal insulin should be adjusted.

carbohydrate content of foods. Unfortunately, this method is not always practical for patients as it does require a higher level of thinking and a more sophisticated knowledge of carbohydrate foods.

The plate method

The plate method is a simplified meal plan that uses a standard 10-inch dinner plate that is divided. One-half of the plate should contain nonstarchy vegetables, one-fourth should contain lean protein, and one-fourth should contain starch. Patients may also choose to have sides of fruit and milk.

Both the constant carbohydrate and carbohydrate counting method rely heavily on food labels, or the "Nutrition Facts." Patients should be cautioned to still learn the meal exchange list, as not every food has a food label and food label information still requires a working knowledge of portion estimation; patients still need to be able to estimate common portions such as half a cup, one cup, etc. An incredible amount of useful nutrition information can be found on the food label with the simple guidelines listed in the next section.

Food labels

- *Serving size*: all information is based on eating the listed serving size.
  - If more or less is eaten, then the patient must calculate this change to the listed nutrients.
  - For example, if portion is ½ cup and provides 15 g of carbohydrate but the patient eats 1 cup, then he or she is actually getting 30 g of carbohydrate.
- *Total carbohydrate*: Includes all forms of carbohydrate (sugar, fiber, sugar alcohols).
- *Fiber*: If there are 5 g of fiber or more, it may be subtracted from the total carbohydrate. If there is less than 5 g of fiber, no action should be taken.
- *Sugar*: Includes naturally occurring and added sugars.
- *Sugar alcohols (polyols)*: Include sorbitol, xylitol, and mannitol.
  - These have about half of the effect of sugar.

- Patients can subtract half of the grams of sugar alcohols from the total carbohydrate.
- Patients should be cautioned that sugar alcohols may cause diarrhea if eaten in excess; the "dose" varies from person to person.
- *Sugar-free* The legal definition is there is less than 0.5 g of sugar per serving, but it does not mean the product is carbohydrate free.
- *No added sugar*: Means there was no sugar added, but it does not mean the product is carbohydrate free.
- *Reduced sugar*: Product has 25% or less sugar than the regular product.
- Alterations in macronutrients:
  - Patients should be cautioned when buying "low carb" and "fat free" products that the calories may be the same or higher than the original version.
  - Food manufacturers may add more fat to "low carb" products and more sugar to "fat free" or low fat products.
- *List of ingredients*: Are done by weight so that the first ingredient is primarily what makes up most of the food.
- *Free foods*: Have less than 20 calories and 5 g of carbohydrate per serving.
- Percent daily values can be useful for general nutrition recommendations:
  - *Fat, cholesterol, and sodium*: Look for 10% or less per serving (remember the serving size and portion consumed do not have to be the same amount).
  - *Micronutrients*: Look for 10% or more for vitamins and minerals.

Macronutrients

The optimal mix of macronutrients should be individualized. Various comorbidities may require that these nutrients be manipulated to better serve the patient's health and disease state.

Carbohydrates

Patients with diabetes no longer have to avoid sugar, but they should be counseled to choose most of their carbohydrate foods from fruits, vegetables, low fat milk or yogurt, and whole grains rather than nutrient-deficient choices such as candy, desserts, and other high-sugar, low-nutrition foods. There does not seem to be any real difference between the the effect of "naturally occurring sugar" and "added sugar" on blood sugar levels. Rather, the total amount of carbohydrate consumed has the largest effect.

Protein

People with diabetes do not require more or less protein than the general population but do benefit from choosing lean or low-fat protein choices. With certain comorbidities, the amount of protein consumed may have to be manipulated to aid the patient's health and disease state.

Table 7.11 Carbohydrate (key points)

- Primarily, the amount of carbohydrate consumed affects blood glucose levels.
- Encourage consumption of fruits, vegetables, whole grains, legumes, and low fat milk to emphasize nutrient-rich, high-fiber foods.
- Macronutrient mix
  - When carbohydrate foods are eaten with protein and/or fat-containing foods, there can be an effect on blood glucose levels.
  - It seems to be advantageous to combine carbohydrate food with protein foods for satiety.
  - High-fat meals can significantly delay gastric emptying and so may affect when the peak postprandial blood sugar level occurs.
- This could have implications with bolused rapid-acting insulin.
- Some patients may benefit from using the glycemic index/glycemic load of foods for a moderate improvement on blood glucose control.
- In general, 60% to 70% of calories should come from carbohydrate and monounsaturated fats. This may be altered to aid with weight loss or to benefit certain lab values and other comorbidities of individual patients.
- Low carbohydrate diets
  - May be beneficial for short-term rapid weight loss compared to traditional meal plans for people with diabetes.
  - This should be determined on an individual basis.
  - Patients should be monitored for any change in blood lipids or any other harmful changes to key lab values.
- Fiber recommendations are no different than for the general population (25 to 35 grams per day).
- Carbohydrates contain 4 calories per gram.

Table 7.12 Protein (key points)

- Even though protein consumption does stimulate insulin release, it does not significantly affect blood sugar levels.
- In general, 10% to 20% of total calories should come from protein.
- If kidneys are normally functioning, there is no need to restrict protein intake.
- Patients with microalbuminuria or nephropathy may benefit from restricting protein to 0.8 to 1.0 g/kg body weight.
- Emphasis should be placed on choosing low-fat protein choices.
- Protein contains 4 calories per gram.

Fat

In general, because dietary fat is such a concentrated source of calories and has a significant influence on cardiovascular disease, it should be limited. Diabetic patients may notice that the rise in postprandial blood sugar may be delayed after eating a high-fat meal. This can be especially problematic for patients on rapid-acting bolus insulin because the rise in blood sugar may not "match" when the insulin is working at its peak.

Table 7.13 Fat (key points)

- Total fat intake usually makes up 30% or less of total calories.
- Patients should be cautioned against eating high-fat meals because of:
  - excess calories.
  - delay in gastric emptying and its subsequent (possible) effect on timing of postprandial blood glucose rise.
- Monounsaturated fats
  - Combined with carbohydrates, foods make up 60% to 70% of calories.
  - Usually alone, make up 10% of total calories.
- Polyunsaturated fats
  - Generally should be 10% or less of total calories.
- Saturated fats
  - Should be limited to no more than 10% of total calories for general health and 7% or less for those individuals with LDL cholesterol above goal.
  - These are among the largest dietary influences on ↑ LDL cholesterol.
- Trans fats
  - Any product with hydrogenated oil.
  - Should be avoided completely if possible.
  - Have a great effect on ↑ LDL and ↓ HDL cholesterol.
- Fat contains 9 calories per gram.

Table 7.14 Dietary cholesterol (key points)

- General recommendations are to keep intake <300 mg/day.
- If LDL above goal, further restricting dietary cholesterol to <200 mg/day may be beneficial.
- Dietary cholesterol does not have as great an effect on blood cholesterol as do saturated and trans fats.

Dietary cholesterol

Dietary cholesterol does not have as large an effect on LDL cholesterol as do saturated and trans fats. General recommendations for dietary cholesterol are to keep intake to less than 300 mg/day.

Other nutrients

- Sodium
  - Sodium goal is ≤2400 mg per day (average American consumes 5 to 6 g Na per day).
  - With nephropathy and hypertension, a restriction of 2000 mg per day may be beneficial.

Micronutrients

- Unless a deficiency exists, there does not seem to be any greater benefit from supplements to patients with diabetes.

Alcohol

- General recommendations: Men no more than 2 drinks per day; women no more than 1 drink per day. One drink is equivalent to 1.5 ounces of distilled alcohol, 4 ounces of wine, or 12 ounces of beer.
- People with diabetes do not need to restrict alcohol consumption any more than the general population does. Great caution should be paid to patients with history of "binge drinking."
- To reduce the likelihood of hypoglycemia, alcohol should only be consumed with meals.
- The caloric impact of alcohol should be emphasized to patients attempting to lose weight (7 calories/gram).

The three main types of diabetes, in general, do not necessitate a different diet approach. One main difference with type 1 diabetes is that all patients must take insulin to manage their blood sugar levels. Patients with type 2 diabetes and gestational diabetes may or may not need insulin. The use of insulin can actually make meal planning much more flexible, as the patient theoretically should be able to "cover" postprandial blood glucose excursions on a meal-by-meal basis. If a patient would like to eat more or less carbohydrate, he or she would take more or less rapid-acting insulin (see section on carbohydrate counting).

Type 1

Diet Rx

- Carbohydrate intake individualized.
  - Ideally, goal is to move patients to carbohydrate counting rather than a fixed meal plan.
  - Alternate methods exist to determine carbohydrate-to-insulin ratio (CIR).
    - One method is starting with 1 unit of rapid-acting insulin for every 15 g carbohydrate and then monitoring preprandial and postprandial blood glucose levels to determine adequacy or need for further titration.

Type 2

Diet Rx

- Usually start patient off on a "fixed meal plan." Depending on patient's treatment plan, he or she may move on to carbohydrate counting.
- Usually requires calorie restriction to aid weight loss.

Gestational diabetes/type 1 or type 2 diabetes and pregnancy

Diet Rx

- Optimize blood glucose levels while avoiding starvation ketosis or ketonemia from ketoacidosis.
- Adjust carbohydrate and caloric intake based on blood sugars, weight gain, and presence or absence of ketosis.
- No different than nondiabetic patients for micronutrients.
- An individualized meal plan including 3 meals and 2 to 4 snacks daily should be provided.
- There may be some benefit to limiting carbohydrate intake during the morning.

References

1. American Association of Diabetes Educators. Definitions; AADE 7™ Self-care Behaviors. Available at: http://www.diabeteseducator.org/ProfessionalResources/AADE7. Accessed April 24, 2008.

2. Funnell M, Brown TL, Childs BP, et al. National standards for diabetes self-management education. *Diabetes Care.* 2007;30:1632.

3. National Institutes of Health and Centers for Disease Control and Prevention (CDC). *Seven Principles for Controlling Your Diabetes for Life.* Atlanta; CDC: 2001. NIH publication No. 99-43431.

4. American Dietetic Association. Definitions in the Medicare MNT benefit proposed regulations: medical nutrition therapy. Available at: http://www.eatright.org/cps/rde/xchg/ada/hs.xsl/nutrition_3391_ENU_HTML.htm. Accessed April 24, 2008.

5. American Diabetes Association. Nutrition recommendations and interventions for diabetes. A position statement of the American Diabetes Association. *Diabetes Care.* 2008;31(suppl 1):S61.

Chapter 8

Insulin therapy in hospitalized patients with diabetes mellitus

Guillermo E. Umpierrez

Hyperglycemia is a frequent manifestation of both critical and noncritical illness, resulting from the acute metabolic and hormonal changes associated with the response to injury and stress. Increasing evidence suggests that in hospitalized patients with and without diabetes, the presence of hyperglycemia is associated with increased risk of complications and death.[1,2] Observational studies among patients with critical illness, acute myocardial infarction, trauma, and/or stroke and patients undergoing coronary artery bypass surgery suggest that aggressive glycemic control positively affects morbidity and mortality. Prospective randomized trials have shown that intense glucose control with continuous insulin infusions in patients with acute critical illness reduces the risk of multiorgan failure and systemic infections and decreases both short- and long-term mortality.[3–5] In addition, improving glycemic control has shown to be cost effective, resulting in significant cost savings.[6]

Goals of glycemic control in the hospital

A recent position statement of the American Association of Clinical Endocrinologists and the American Diabetes Association recommended glycemic targets between 80 and 110 mg/dL for critical patients in the intensive care unit (ICU).[7] For patients with noncritical illness, a preprandial blood glucose less than 110 mg/dL and a random blood glucose level less than 180 mg/dL were recommended. Recently, several groups have raised concerns about these recommendations, and higher target glucose levels have been recommended[8,9] (Table 8.1). Because of concerns of hypoglycemia and its effect on hospital morbidity and mortality reported in recent observational randomized clinical trials,[10–12] more conservative glucose targets have been recommended in the ICU.[8,9] Based on an extensive review of published clinical trials in critical and noncritical ill patients, the advisable in-hospital targets are to maintain fasting and preprandial glucose levels between 90 and 140 mg/dL, respectively, and a random glucose level less than 180 mg/dL.

Table 8.1 In-hospital glycemic targets

	ICU	Non-ICU	
		Fasting BG	Random BG
AACE	≤110	≤110	≤180
ADA	≤110	90 to 130	≤180
AHA	90 to 140		<180
EU	80 to 130	<140	<180

AACE, American Association of Clinical Endocrinology (ref); ADA, American Diabetes Association; AHA, American Heart Association; BG, blood glucose; EU, Emory University School of Medicine (metabolism); ICU, intensive care unit.

Monitoring glycemic control

Success of any regimen requires frequent blood glucose monitoring to allow early detection of any alterations in metabolic control. The frequency of bedside glucose testing should be determined by the patient's condition and specific situations. During continuous insulin infusion, capillary blood glucose should be measured every hour until blood glucose is within goal range for about 4 hours, and then measurement can be decreased to every 2 hours. In the non–intensive care setting and in patients receiving subcutaneous insulin therapy, bedside glucose testing should be performed before each meal and at bedtime.

Even though knowing the glycemic control in the period preceding the hospital admission rarely influences the acute management of diabetes, measuring Hb_{A1c} levels is of great importance to make plans at discharge and for the outpatient management of diabetes. If the glycemic control has been poor and the circumstances allow it, the patient can have a one-on-one session with the nutritionist and diabetes educator. So if the patient has not had this measurement done in the month preceding the admission or the results are not available, the Hb_{A1c} should be measured.

Use of oral antidiabetic agents in the hospital

The safety and efficacy of oral antidiabetic agents in hospitalized patients have not been established; however, there are major limitations to the use of these agents in the hospital setting, including the slow onset of action, inability to make rapid dose adjustments in response to changing inpatient needs, and the risk of hypoglycemia. In addition, each oral agent has its own contraindications that may limit its use. A long-standing controversy exists regarding the vascular effects of sulfonylureas in patients with cardiac and cerebral ischemia. Data suggest that they may inhibit ischemic preconditioning and predispose to vascular events. A large number of patients have one or more contraindications to the use of metformin, including congestive heart failure, renal dysfunction, or liver dysfunction.[2] Thiazolidinediones increase intravascular volume and may precipitate or worsen congestive heart failure, peripheral edema, and ischemic events.

Because of these limitations and the lack of safety and efficacy data from prospective randomized clinical trials, the use of oral agents cannot be recommended in the hospital setting.

Continuous insulin infusion algorithms

Insulin is the preferred and more effective agent for achieving and maintaining glucose control in the hospital. The insulin dose and route of administration are decided based on the type of diabetes, nature and extent of the medical or surgical illness, antecedent pharmacological therapy, and state of metabolic control.[13]

Indications for the use of continuous intravenous infusion (CII) administration (Table 8.2) include diabetic ketoacidosis and hyperosmolar hyperglycemic state, intraoperative and postoperative care, the postoperative period following heart surgery and organ transplantation, acute myocardial infarction, stroke, and critical care illness.[2,14] During critical illness, patients may experience significant changes of insulin requirements, peripheral edema, impaired perfusion of subcutaneous sites, requirement for pressor support, and/or use of total parenteral nutrition. In these settings, CII has been shown to be superior to the subcutaneous injection of insulin with respect to rapidity of effect in controlling hyperglycemia, overall ability to achieve glycemic control, and, most important, preventing hypoglycemic episodes. These algorithms aim to achieve correction of hyperglycemia in a timely manner and determine the insulin infusion rate required to maintain blood sugars within a defined target range.

A variety of CII algorithms have been reported in the literature.[3,4,15,16] These algorithms can be grouped into two major types: fixed and dynamic insulin infusion rates. Tables 8.3 and 8.4 describe examples of fixed rate and dynamic drip algorithms used at our institution. In brief, fixed rate algorithms recommend changes on the infusion rate based solely on the patient's current blood glucose value. Although they are easy to implement, limitations of the fixed rate algorithms are that changes in insulin doses do not take into consideration previous values or the slope of glucose change during treatment and do not take into account differences in insulin sensitivity among patients. Dynamic algorithms overcome these deficiencies by taking into consideration current blood glucose level, the rate of change in blood glucose, and insulin sensitivity.[17] Recently, results of

Table 8.2 Indications for intravenous insulin therapy in subjects with hyperglycemia

- Critical illness
- Perioperative period
- Prolonged NPO (nothing by mouth) status
- Diabetic ketoacidosis
- Hyperosmolar hyperglycemic syndrome
- Total parenteral nutrition therapy
- Labor and delivery
- Other acute medical or surgical illnesses requiring prompt glucose control

Table 8.3 Perioperative management of patients with diabetes

I. Surgery in type 2 diabetic patients *not* treated with insulin: Minor surgery

- Hold oral agents the day of surgery
- Patients with "fair" metabolic control (fasting blood glucose <180 mg/dL): cover with regular or rapid-acting (lispro, aspart, glulisine) insulin as needed (see Table 8.5)
- Patients with "poor" metabolic control (fasting blood glucose >180 mg/dL): start continuous insulin infusion
- *Goals*: avoid excessive hyperglycemia (blood glucose >180 mg/dL) and hypoglycemia (blood glucose <80 mg/dL)

II. Surgery in type 1 and type 2 diabetic patients *treated* with insulin: Minor surgery

- Hold oral agents the day of surgery
- Patients in "fair" metabolic control (fasting blood glucose <180 mg/dL):
  - Give ½ of intermediate-acting insulin (NPH) the morning of the surgery
  - While NPO, infuse dextrose 5% saline plus KCl (10 to 20 mEq/L) at 100 mL/h
  - Check blood glucose every 4 to 6 hours while NPO and supplement with short-acting insulin as needed
  - Patient treated with basal insulin analogues (glargine, detemir) should receive 80% to 100% of their usual basal insulin dose; similarly, patients treated with continuous insulin infusion therapy (insulin pump) should receive their usual basal infusion rate
  - Restart preadmission insulin therapy once food intake is tolerated
  - Patients in "poor" control—fasting blood glucose >180 mg/dL, start continuous insulin infusion

III. Surgery in type 1 and type 2 diabetic patients *treated* with insulin: Major surgery

- Hold oral agents the day of surgery
- Start continuous insulin infusion prior to surgery and continue during perioperative period
- *Goals*: Maintain blood glucose <180 mg/dL during surgery and blood glucose between 80 and 140 mg/dL during the perioperative period in the surgical intensive care unit. Start subcutaneous insulin two hours prior to discontinuation of insulin infusion. In non–intensive care unit settings, avoid excessive hyperglycemia (blood glucose >180 mg/dL) and hypoglycemia (blood glucose <80 mg/dL)

Conversion factors to SI units: serum glucose (mg/dL) × 0.055 mmol/L.

several electronic versions of dynamic insulin drip algorithms have become available in Europe and the United States. We recently compared the results of a randomized control trial comparing the efficacy and safety of a computer-guided (Glucommander) versus a standard paper form in critically ill patients in the ICU. The mean blood glucose was significantly lower in patients treated with the computer-based algorithm (103 ± 9 mg/dL) than those treated with the standard paper form protocol (117 ± 9 mg/dL, $p < 0.001$). In addition, the use of the computer-based protocol was associated with a shorter time to achieve the study blood glucose target of 80 to 120 mg/dL and less glucose variability during the drip infusion, as shown by a greater percentage of glucose measurements maintained within target. The computer-based algorithm, however, resulted in a higher risk of mild hypoglycemic events and required more frequent glucose testing than did the standard protocol. Of interest, no differences were observed in mortality, ICU length of stay, or hospital length of stay between treatment groups.

Table 8.4 Insulin regimens in non-ICU settings

A. Basal Bolus Insulin Regimen

- Basal insulin: glargine and detemir
- Bolus or prandial insulin: lispro, aspart, glulisine

Patients treated with diet and/or or oral agents (insulin naive) prior to admission

- Hold oral antidiabetic drugs
- Starting total daily insulin dose:
  - 0.4 unit per kilogram of body weight per day when blood glucose concentration is between 140 and 200 mg/dL
  - 0.5 unit per kilogram of body weight per day when blood glucose concentration is between 201 and 400 mg/dL
  - Lower insulin doses (0.3 unit per kilogram of body weight per day) should be given to elderly patients and/or patients with renal failure (GFR <60 mL/min)
- Half of total daily dose will be given as basal insulin and half as rapid-acting insulin.
- Give basal insulin once daily, at the same time of the day.
- Rapid-acting insulin should be given in three equally divided doses before each meal. Hold rapid-acting insulin if a patient is not able to eat to prevent hypoglycemia.

Patients treated with insulin prior to admission

- Insulin-treated patients should be started at the same amount of outpatient insulin dose.
- Half of total daily dose will be given as basal insulin and half as rapid-acting insulin.
- Basal insulin should be given once daily, at the same time of the day.
- Rapid-acting insulin should be given in three equally divided doses before each meal. Hold rapid-acting insulin if a patient is not able to eat to prevent hypoglycemia.
- Supplemental insulin: supplemental doses of rapid-acting insulin to correct hyperglycemia (see Table 8.5).
- Insulin adjustment
  - If fasting and premeal BG <140 mg/dL (in the absence of hypoglycemia): no change
  - If fasting and premeal BG between 140 and 180 mg/dL (in the absence of hypoglycemia): increase basal insulin by 10% every day.
  - If fasting and premeal BG >180 mg/dL in the absence of hypoglycemia: increase basal insulin dose by 20%.
  - If hypoglycemia (<70 mg/dL), decrease total daily insulin dose by 20%.

B. NPH and regular insulin twice daily

Patients treated with diet and/or oral agents (insulin naive) prior to admission

- Hold oral antidiabetic drugs on admission.
- Starting total daily insulin dose:
  - 0.4 unit per kilogram of body weight per day when the admission and/or mean blood glucose concentration is between 140 and 200 mg/dL
  - 0.5 unit per kilogram of body weight per day when the admission and/or mean blood glucose concentration is between 201 and 400 mg/dL
- Two-thirds of the total daily dose is given in the morning and one-third in the evening.
- The morning and evening insulin dose are given as two-thirds NPH and one-third regular insulin.
- Hold regular insulin if a patient is not able to eat to prevent hypoglycemia.

Table 8.4 (*Contd.*)

Patients treated with insulin prior to admission

• Subjects receiving NPH insulin plus regular insulin should be started at the outpatient insulin schedule and dosage.

• Two-thirds of the total daily dose is given in the morning and one-third in the evening.

• The insulin dose is given as two-thirds NPH and one-third regular insulin.

• Hold regular insulin if a patient is not able to eat to prevent hypoglycemia.

Supplemental insulin: supplemental doses of regular insulin (see Table 8.5)

• Insulin adjustment

• If fasting and premeal BG <140 mg/dL (in the absence of hypoglycemia): no change.

• If fasting and premeal BG between 140 and 180 mg/dL (in the absence of hypoglycemia): increase total insulin dose by 10% every day.

• If fasting and premeal BG >180 mg/dL in the absence of hypoglycemia: increase total insulin dose by 20%.

• If hypoglycemia (<70 mg/dL), decrease total daily insulin dose by 20%.

Glycemic control in non-ICU settings

The importance of glycemic control is not limited to patients in critical care areas and may also apply to patients admitted to general surgical and medical wards. In such patients, the development of hyperglycemia in those with or without a history of diabetes has been associated with prolonged hospital stay, infections, disability after hospital discharge, and death.[3–5,17] In general surgical patients, a serum glucose greater than 220 mg/dL on postoperative day 1 has been shown to be a sensitive, albeit nonspecific, predictor of the development of serious postoperative hospital-acquired infection.[18] A retrospective review of 1886 admissions to a community hospital in Atlanta, Georgia, found an 18-fold increase in mortality in hyperglycemic patients without a history of diabetes and a 2.5-fold increase in mortality in patients with known diabetes compared with controls.[1] More recently, hyperglycemia on admission was also shown to be independently associated with adverse outcomes in patients with community-acquired pneumonia.[19] Our protocol for the management of diabetes in non critical patients[20] is outlined in Table 8.4, and general guidelines for the management of patients during the perioperative period is outlined in Table 8.5.

Effective insulin therapy must provide both basal and nutritional meals in order to achieve the target goals. Hospitalized patients often require high insulin doses to achieve target glucose levels due to increased insulin resistance; thus, in addition to basal and nutritional insulin requirements, patients often require supplemental or correction insulin for treatment of hyperglycemia. Use of "sliding scale" insulin alone is discouraged; evidence does not support this technique because it has resulted in unacceptably high rates of hyperglycemia, hypoglycemia, and iatrogenic diabetic ketoacidosis in hospitalized patients. We recently reported the results of a prospective, multicenter randomized trial to compare the efficacy and safety of a basal/bolus insulin regimen to sliding scale regular insulin (SSI) in patients with type 2 diabetes (RABBIT 2 trial).[20] A total of 130 insulin-naive patients were randomized to receive glargine and glulisine or the sliding scale protocol. Glargine was given once daily and glulisine was given before meals at a starting dose of 0.4 unit/kg/day for blood glucose 140 to 200 mg/dL or 0.5 unit/kg/day for blood glucose 201 to 400 mg/dL. SSI was given 4 times/day for blood glucose >140 mg/dL (Table 8.4). We observed that treatment with basal bolus insulin regimen resulted in a significant improvement in glycemic control compared to the sole use of SSI. The mean daily glucose difference between groups ranged from 23 to 58 mg/dL during days 2–6 of therapy. A blood glucose target of <140 mg/dL was achieved in two-thirds of patients treated with insulin glargine and glulisine, whereas only one-third of those treated with SSI achieved target glycemia. Despite increasing insulin doses, one-fifth of patients treated with SSI had persistently elevated glucose levels >240 mg/dL during the hospital stay. In such patients, glycemic control rapidly improved after switching to the basal/bolus insulin regimen. Based on these results, we conclude that a basal/bolus insulin regimen is preferred over SSI alone in the management of non–critically ill patients with type 2 diabetes.

More recently, we reported the results of a randomized controlled trial comparing the safety and efficacy of a basal bolus insulin regimen with insulin detemir and aspart insulin to a standard split mixed regimen of NPH and regular insulin in patients with type 2 diabetes. A total of 130 nonsurgical patients with blood glucose levels between 140 and 400 mg/dL were assigned to receive either detemir once daily and aspart before meals or NPH and regular twice daily. Total daily dose (TDD) was started at 0.4 unit/kg/day for blood glucose 140 to 200 mg/dL or 0.5 unit/kg/day for blood glucose 201 to 400 mg/dL. We observed that the mean daily blood glucose level during therapy, the number of blood glucose readings within target (<140 mg/dL), and the number of hypoglycemic episodes were not different between the two treatment regimens. We concluded that the basal/bolus regimen with detemir once daily and aspart before meals results in equivalent glycemic control compared with a split-mixed regimen of NPH and regular in hospitalized patients with type 2 diabetes.

Risk of hypoglycemia

Tight glycemic control can result in increased rate of hypoglycemic events in hospitalized patients.[9] The incidence of hypoglycemia in published trials of tight glycemic control has varied, because of differences among the types of patients enrolled in clinical trials, differences in blood glucose values defining hypoglycemia, type of glucose monitoring, and the intensity of the intervention. The rate of severe hypoglycemia, defined as glucose level <40 mg/dL, has ranged between 5% and 18.7% of patients in different ICU trials.[10,21] Of interest, higher rates have been observed in medical ICU patients compared with surgical patients. Case-control series and randomized clinical trials have reported that severe hypoglycemia does not independently increase the risk of mortality.[4,11] In more recent trials, however, severe hypoglycemia was found to be an independent factor for increased risk of mortality.[4,11] This is a concern in critically ill, noncommunicating, and sedated patients with mechanical ventilation in whom detection of hypoglycemia requires frequent accurate glucose monitoring.

Despite exciting findings of a decrease in mortality in critically ill patients with the use of tight glucose control and the restoration of normal values of blood glucose through intensive insulin therapy, two recent European multicenter randomized clinical trials—VISEP and GLUCONTROL—raised clinically important concerns regarding the safety and efficacy of tight glycemic control in critically ill patients; moreover, both studies failed to confirm the data of the Leuven group.[10,12] The VISEP trial was stopped after the inclusion of 488 patients in 17 centers, for safety reasons (i.e., a large increase in the rate of hypoglycemia) and lack of efficacy (i.e., no significant difference in the 28- or the 90-day mortality rates).[12] Similarly, the enrollment of patients in GLUCONTROL was stopped prematurely because of the occurrence of severe hypoglycemia without concurrent improvement in survival. In this study, subjects were randomized to a blood glucose target between 140 and 180 mg/dL or between 80 and 110 mg/dL. The rates of hypoglycemia and mortality in the patients having experienced at least one episode of severe hypoglycemia (defined as a blood glucose <40 mg/dL) were both higher in the group randomized to the 80 to 110 mg/dL target. These data suggest that a target blood glucose level of between 140 and 180 mg/dL may be safer than a target of 80 to 110 mg/dL. Moreover, as no significant difference in mortality was noted between the two groups, the risk-to-benefit ratio may favor a higher glucose target. Recognized risk factors for hypoglycemia during intensive insulin therapy are severe infections and sepsis and the presence of hepatic, adrenal, or renal failure. In addition, an increased incidence of hypoglycemia has been reported in females and in patients with (1) preexisting diabetes, (2) use of continuous hemofiltration, (3) a lowering of the infusion rate of nutrition without adjustment of the insulin infusion rate, and/or (4) the administration of insulin by itself.

Table 8.5 Protocol for short-acting insulin supplements			
Blood glucose (mg/dL)	**Insulin sensitive**	**Usual**	**Insulin resistant**
>141 to 180	2	4	6
181 to 220	4	6	8
221 to 260	6	8	10
261 to 300	8	10	12
301 to 350	10	12	14
351 to 400	12	14	16
>400	14	16	18

Measure blood glucose before each meal and at bedtime (or every 6 hours if patient not eating). Give full dose before meals and half-dose at bedtime.

Discharge recommendations

Diabetes education should be provided to all patients with newly diagnosed diabetes, and the outpatient treatment regimen should be discussed prior to discharge. The patient, or caregiver, should receive appropriate instruction on proper dietary therapy and on home glucose monitoring techniques. It is important to make the necessary arrangements to ensure appropriate follow-up with a health care professional who will oversee the patient's diabetes management during follow-up. In addition, patients should be educated on the signs and symptoms of hypoglycemia and hyperglycemia and on "sick day" management, including the importance of insulin administration during an illness, blood glucose goals, and the use of supplemental short- or rapid-acting insulin.

References

1. Umpierrez GE, Isaacs SD, Bazargan N, You X, Thaler LM, Kitabchi AE. Hyperglycemia: an independent marker of in-hospital mortality in patients with undiagnosed diabetes. *J Clin Endocrinol Metab.* 2002;87:978–982.

2. Clement S, Braithwaite SS, Magee MF, et al. Management of diabetes and hyperglycemia in hospitals. *Diabetes Care.* 2004;27:553–597.

3. van den Berghe G, Wouters P, Weekers F, et al. Intensive insulin therapy in the critically ill patients. *N Engl J Med.* 2001;345:1359–1367.

4. van den Berghe G, Wilmer A, Hermans G, et al. Intensive insulin therapy in the medical ICU. *N Engl J Med.* 2006;354:449–461.

5. Furnary AP, Gao G, Grunkemeier GL, et al. Continuous insulin infusion reduces mortality in patients with diabetes undergoing coronary artery bypass grafting. *J Thorac Cardiovasc Surg.* 2003;125:1007–1021.

6. Krinsley JS, Jones RL. Cost analysis of intensive glycemic control in critically ill adult patients. *Chest.* 2006;129:644–650.

7. Garber AJ, Moghissi ES, Bransome ED Jr, et al. American College of Endocrinology position statement on inpatient diabetes and metabolic control. *Endocr Pract.* 2004;10(suppl 2):4–9.

8. Deedwania P, Kosiborod M, Barrett E, et al. Hyperglycemia and acute coronary syndrome: a scientific statement from the American Heart Association Diabetes Committee of the Council on Nutrition, Physical Activity, and Metabolism. *Circulation.* 2008;117:1610–1619.

9. Kitabchi AE, Freire AX, Umpierrez GE. Evidence for strict inpatient blood glucose control: time to revise glycemic goals in hospitalized patients. *Metabolism.* 2008;57:116–120.

10. Preiser JC, Brunkhorst F. Tight glucose control and hypoglycemia. *Crit Care Med.* 2008;36:1391–1392.

11. Krinsley JS, Grover A. Severe hypoglycemia in critically ill patients: risk factors and outcomes. *Crit Care Med.* 2007;35:2262–2267.

12. Brunkhorst FM, Engel C, Bloos F, et al. Intensive insulin therapy and pentastarch resuscitation in severe sepsis. *N Engl J Med.* 2008;358:125–139.

13. Smiley DD, Umpierrez GE. Perioperative glucose control in the diabetic or nondiabetic patient. *South Med J.* 2006;99:580–589; quiz 590–591.

14. Umpierrez GE, Kitabshi AE. ICU care for patients with diabetes. *Curr Opin Endocrinol*. 2004;11:75–81.

15. Goldberg PA, Siegel MD, Sherwin RS, et al. Implementation of a safe and effective insulin infusion protocol in a medical intensive care unit. *Diabetes Care*. 2004;27:461–467.

16. Furnary AP, Zerr KJ, Grunkemeier GL, Starr A. Continuous intravenous insulin infusion reduces the incidence of deep sternal wound infection in diabetic patients after cardiac surgical procedures. *Ann Thorac Surg*. 1999;67:352–360; discussion 360–362.

17. Inzucchi SE. Clinical practice. Management of hyperglycemia in the hospital setting. *N Engl J Med*. 2006;355:1903–1911.

18. Pomposelli JJ, Baxter JK 3rd, Babineau TJ, et al. Early postoperative glucose control predicts nosocomial infection rate in diabetic patients. *JPEN J Parenter Enteral Nutr*. 1998;22:77–81.

19. McAlister FA, Majumdar SR, Blitz S, Rowe BH, Romney J, Marrie TJ. The relation between hyperglycemia and outcomes in 2,471 patients admitted to the hospital with community-acquired pneumonia. *Diabetes Care*. 2005;28:810–815.

20. Umpierrez GE, Smiley D, Zisman A, et al. Randomized study of basal-bolus insulin therapy in the inpatient management of patients with type 2 diabetes (RABBIT 2 trial). *Diabetes Care*. 2007;30:2181–2186.

21. Krinsley JS, Preiser JC. Moving beyond tight glucose control to safe effective glucose control. *Crit Care*. 2008;12:149.

Index

99

CPSIA information can be obtained at www.ICGtesting.com
232815LV00004B/2/P